THE ART of CAREGIVING

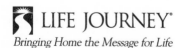
LIFE JOURNEY®

Bringing Home the Message for Life

COOK COMMUNICATIONS MINISTRIES
Colorado Springs, Colorado • Paris, Ontario
KINGSWAY COMMUNICATIONS LTD
Eastbourne, England

Other books by Michael S. Barry

A REASON FOR HOPE
Gaining Strength for Your Fight Against Cancer

A SEASON FOR HOPE
Daily Encouragement for Your Fight Against Cancer

THE ART of CAREGIVING

HOW TO LEND SUPPORT & ENCOURAGEMENT TO THOSE WITH CANCER

MICHAEL S. BARRY

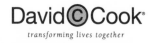
David C Cook®

transforming lives together

THE ART OF CAREGIVING
Published by David C. Cook
4050 Lee Vance View
Colorado Springs, CO 80918 U.S.A.

David C. Cook Distribution Canada
55 Woodslee Avenue, Paris, Ontario, Canada N3L 3E5

David C. Cook U.K., Kingsway Communications
Eastbourne, East Sussex BN23 6NT, England

The Web site addresses recommended throughout this book are
offered as a resource to you. These Web sites are not intended
in any way to be or imply an endorsement on the part of Cook
Communications Ministries, nor do we vouch for their content.

All Scripture quotations, unless otherwise noted, are taken
from the *Holy Bible, New International Version®. NIV®.*
Copyright © 1973, 1978, 1984 by International Bible Society.
Used by permission of Zondervan. All rights reserved.
Scripture quotations marked MSG are taken from *THE
MESSAGE.* Copyright © by Eugene H. Peterson 1993, 1994,
1995, 1996, 2000, 2001, 2002. Used by permission of
NavPress Publishing Group; and KJV are from the King James
Version of the Bible. (Public Domain.) Italics in quotations have
been added by the author for emphasis.

ISBN 978-0-7814-4430-9
LCCN 2007921062

Cover Photo: © 2007 iStockPhoto
Cover Design: ThinkPen Design, llc

First printing, 2007
Printed in Canada

2 3 4 5 6 7 8 9 10

091008

To
Helen Wade Buescher,
caring wife of Jack Buescher,
caring daughter of Riley and Helen Wyatt,
caring sister of Miles Wyatt
and sister-in-law Jane Wyatt,
caring aunt of my wife, Kay, and her sister, Joy,
caring great-aunt to my daughters, Sara and Becca,
and who may never know
how much I admire her
and appreciate her generous heart
or the hopeful joy
her candle has brought to so many,
including me

ALL THE DARKNESS IN THE UNIVERSE CANNOT
EXTINGUISH THE LIGHT OF A SINGLE CANDLE.
— ANCIENT PROVERB

Contents

Caregiving is an art, one more demanding than sculpting, painting, or writing poetry—and it's potentially more rewarding, too. Yet those who are called to practice this art rarely have the experience or education to guide them. Cancer is a diagnosis that often creates fear and turns lives upside down, sometimes more for loved ones than for the individual given the diagnosis. My friend and colleague Rev. Dr. Michael Barry uses his extensive experience, education, and innate talent to serve as mentor and understanding teacher—an artist's guide, if you will—for those providing care to those who are ill. Though focused on caregivers of cancer patients, these principles are equally appropriate for caregivers supporting loved ones through any disabling, intensive, or life-threatening condition.

Through years of ministering to the needs of cancer patients and their loved ones, Michael has developed a unique philosophy of caregiving, which he shares in this book along with numerous insider tips that you will find invaluable. He provides insights into principles described by psychologists as "flow"—the optimum emotional experience sometimes referred to as "in the zone"—woven with the biblical concept of joy. The timeless principles that Michael draws from Scripture are equally applicable to people of all faiths. Even more importantly, the wisdom he offers provides a framework for experiencing inner joy regardless of circumstances.

I have had the privilege of working closely with Michael in Philadelphia, Pennsylvania, as we have shared in the rare experience of founding a new cancer hospital. Together, with a few other very carefully chosen colleagues, we shared the incredible gift of purpose provided freely by patients and their loved ones as they seek options for hope and healing that they can find nowhere else. I have repeatedly seen Michael lead caregivers through mysteries unlocked, facilitating powerful transformations and creating a healing environment for caregivers and patient alike.

Caregiving is more than an act of love; effective caregiving is an *art* of love. Now, through *The Art of Caregiving*, Michael helps you bypass the awkward stumbling of one who is called upon to perform a difficult art without experience. With Michael's help, you, too, can unlock the mysteries and develop your own "art of caregiving," experiencing joy, flow, and the highest quality of life possible when you need it most.

JOHN M. MCNEIL

President and Chief Executive Officer

Cancer Treatment Centers of America at Eastern Regional Medical Center

Opening the Door

― ❖ ―

BEST FRIEND, MY WELL-SPRING IN THE WILDERNESS!

—George Eliot

I WILL STAY ON AT EPHESUS UNTIL PENTECOST,
BECAUSE A GREAT DOOR FOR EFFECTIVE WORK HAS OPENED TO ME.

—1 Corinthians 16:8–9

I admire you and your willingness to help your loved one battle a mean disease. I appreciate your courage as well. But most importantly, I thank you for your help. You are, or can be, one of the greatest weapons in your loved one's fight against cancer. Did you know that "within the health-care industry, it is becoming widely recognized that family members, close friends, and 'significant others' can have a far greater impact on patients' experience of illness, and on their long-term health and happiness, than any health-care professional"?[1] That's because you're often at the front line of defense initiating medical care and also shoring up the rear guard by ensuring that your friend or loved one receives dignified care and protection. Those of us in the health-care field want to acknowledge your significance and applaud you for your courage, as well as welcome you to the health-care team. We appreciate you and value your commitment and love.

I've written this book to empower you to be a "candle of joyful hope" to your loved one whose life has been darkened by cancer. Cancer treatment is often a nighttime journey through a wilderness in which patients and their caregivers are confronted with worry and fear, a journey in which the slightest flicker of hope means more than words can express. And you, with God's help, will be that flicker of hope. You can do this. This book will be a candle of hope for you.

We know you need more than information to be an effective beacon of joyful hope—you also need emotional support. My prayer is that through this book you might sense my heart touching yours and that you'll discover you are not alone in your struggle to hang in there with your loved one; there are many, many others who are hanging in there with you.

Caregiving often has emotional highs and lows. In this book I will share some of the ways some health-care professionals minimize moments of sadness, low energy, and depression. I will teach you a philosophy of caregiving that creates high energy and engenders a life-giving and joyful attitude, even amid great difficulty.

Helen Keller said, "When one door of happiness closes, another opens; but often we look so long at the closed door that we do not see the one which has been opened for us."[2]

Too many caregivers, including health-care professionals, look at the "closed door." In honor of you as a caregiver, I dedicate this book to God, who always provides an open door for those who patiently wait for him. Perhaps this book is the key to the door you've been waiting to see open. As you read, may you sense that a great door for effective work has opened for you.

However, you will not be the caregiver you need to be by your own strength. In fact, it is hopeless. The tasks are too difficult, and the expectations are too high. Only those who understand their "hopelessness" will receive the power and strength from God that is needed to help carry the cross of someone they love. As the Lord teaches, we do well to remember, "I am the vine; you are the branches. If a man remains in me and I in him, he will bear much fruit; apart from me you can do nothing" (John 15:5).

MICHAEL S. BARRY
PHILADELPHIA, PENNSYLVANIA

CHAPTER ONE

A Privilege and a Challenge

---❖---

WISDOM IS SUPREME; THEREFORE GET WISDOM.
THOUGH IT COST ALL YOU HAVE, GET UNDERSTANDING.

—Proverbs 4:7

Most cancer patients and caregivers are quietly frantic; they hunger for solid and dependable advice. A few minutes in the cafeteria of a cancer hospital will convince you of that. Patients and their caregivers often sit with other patients and their caregivers, sharing their experiences and giving advice about what seems to help or work and what doesn't. Further, the information available on cancer and caregiving through the local bookstore or the Internet is endless. This book is different in that it allows you to enter into the mind of a Christian pastor and chaplain who ministers to and counsels cancer patients and their caregivers every day all day long. What I have to share that is perhaps somewhat unique is my philosophy of caregiving, a philosophy that can be applied to various caregiving situations and is based on the biblical concept of joy.

I take seriously Psalm 118:24: "This is the day the LORD has made; let us rejoice and be glad in it." Why should we rejoice today?

Because not one of us knows how long we are going to live. Today is the only day we know we have, so why not live joyfully?

There is a practical side to my philosophy, though. It is not only biblical; it also serves as a counterbalance to the difficulties we all face in our attempts to help a loved one survive a disease. Here's some of what I know about you:

YOU WOULD DO IT ANYWAY

The diagnosis of cancer in a loved one creates feelings of fear and anxiety, but even more common is the feeling of desperation. Soon thereafter we are visited by the unwanted and uninvited feelings of anger, hopelessness, despair, and sheer exhaustion. As unwelcome as these feelings are, and as much as you might like to hand over the caregiving to someone else, truth be known, you would do it anyway, the weariness and difficulty notwithstanding. Consider the following statistics based on a survey done by the University of Pennsylvania Family Caregiver Cancer Education Program.

CANCER CAREGIVER'S PROFILE:

82% are female.

71% are married.

61% have been providing care for less than six months.

54% live with the patient for whom they are caring.

47% are more than 50 years old.

36% reported that caregiving required more than 40 hours of time per week.

PHYSICAL PROBLEMS THEY ENCOUNTERED:

70% reported taking between 1 and 10 medications per day.

62% reported their own health had suffered as a result of caregiving.

25% reported having significant physical limitations of their own.

EMOTIONAL PROBLEMS THEY ENCOUNTERED:

85% reported that they resented having to provide care.

70% reported that their families were not working well together.

54% reported that they visited friends and family less since
assuming their caregiving role.

35% reported that they were overwhelmed by their caregiving role.

CONCLUSION:

97% said their roles were important.

**81% said they wanted to provide care and could not live with
themselves if they did not assume caregiving responsibilities.**

67% said they enjoyed providing care.

In spite of the personal suffering, time and energy expended, and
risk to your own physical well-being, the truth is *you would do it
anyway!* What does this say about you? It says you are kind, compassionate, and caring. Further, it says you are willing to assume responsibility for the well-being of another person at a time when that
person is very vulnerable. You are the Good Samaritan. You are
exhibiting selfless love, giving, in part, your life for the sake of
another. In no small measure, you are walking as Jesus walked (1 John
2:6). Your role is important, and so are you! But here's the point: If
you are going to do it anyway, why not allow joy to lighten your
burden and enhance your personal happiness along the way?

You've walked into a situation that many in the world are walking
away from. You obviously care a great deal about someone who is ill. I
understand what you are going through. I have many times walked
the road you are traveling. I want to congratulate you on your
courage. Walking into a difficult situation while others are walking out
is an amazing act of sacrificial love.

But your choice to care for your loved one, whether a selfless
act of love or a decision forced on you by necessity or perhaps
something in between, doesn't mean you're prepared to give quality
care. You may feel woefully inadequate to help your friend. You may
be frightened, depressed, or angry that cancer happened to your
loved one and you. You may never have needed to play a caregiving
role—and it may seem foreign to you. Or you may have played this

role too many times and are weary and grieved about going through it again.

Nonetheless, here you are. The good news is you're taking on a role that can help both you and your loved one grow spiritually, emotionally, and even physically. This is a time you both may come to see as a blessing, one of the best times of your lives. What I offer you is one way of caring for others—a model for engaging a role that you feel called to perform but may feel unprepared or inadequate to assume. You may have never been sick a day in your life and there-fore don't know how it feels to need someone. Maybe you haven't had a good role model to show you how to take care of someone who is ill.

I don't presume you have any experience as a caregiver, though you might have far more experience than I. I simply am making a case for engaging in one particular model of caregiving that I have found helpful.

MY BEST ADVICE FOR YOU

Cancer is like being caught in an undertow. Upon realizing that they are in danger, people usually panic and think, *I'm going to die!* Furiously they try to swim to shore. However, according to the experts, they are the ones least likely to live. Consider this advice.

> When caught in a rip current [undertow], one should not fight it, but rather swim parallel to the shoreline in order to leave it. If you see a person caught in one, yell at them to do so. *Floating* until the current disperses into deeper waters is another method of surviving such a dangerous incident, but it may leave the swimmer farther out from shore.[1]

Floating until the current disperses into deeper water? Sounds crazy, doesn't it? Allowing the wave to take you further away from the shore? And yet, that is what survival requires of us. How is that any different than faithfully trusting in God? During the undertow times in our lives, our human nature is to panic and struggle, when actually just the opposite will help us overcome our problems.

The expert advice is, "If you see a person caught in one, yell at them to do so." OK, so I'm now "yelling" at *you*. Calm down. Lie on your back, so to speak. Allow God to care for you. Trust him. Don't panic, even though it makes sense to do so. The ocean's pull might seem to take you away from safety, but it creates your best chance for survival. Trust God. Now go yell the same advice to your loved one.

THE GOAL OF CAREGIVING

The goal of caregiving is to help your loved one thrive during the process of cancer treatment as well as after, without compromising your own health and well-being. Your goal is not to heal. God does that. You are not God. The doctors are not God. All any of us can do is offer our best to comfort, support, love, and care. If we do that, at the end of every day we will be able to put our heads on our pillows knowing that, our limitations notwithstanding, we did the best possible job to help relieve suffering and inject joy into the life of our loved one.

Cancer patients and their caregivers have much to learn from this story about heart patients:

> Not everyone in Cardiac Rehab [looked fearful and anxiety ridden]. About one-third of the group came in every day looking as though they'd just won the lottery: They'd looked death in the eye—and survived! ...
>
> Every afternoon, all the Phase Three Rehab guys worked out on our various exercise machines.... I came to think of the two groups as the Happy Guys, who were in love with life, and the Scared Guys, who just hated the idea of death. One thing quickly became obvious: Virtually all of the Happy Guys were on the cusp of recovery, with ruddy cheeks, good endurance, and strong numbers on their cardiac health indices. But most of the Scared Guys were ghostly and tentative, with weak numbers.... I realized

that there was something happy people know that unhappy people don't: No matter what happens in life, there's always something left to love, and the love that remains is always stronger than anything that goes against it.[2]

Cancer patients neatly fall into these same categories—happy or scared—with the same general results. Helping you and your loved one learn how to be one of the "happy guys" is really what this book is all about.

The hospital I am proud to represent adheres to what we call the "Mother Standard," which is our way of saying we are to treat all patients as if they were as near and dear to us as our own mothers. We do our best to accomplish this goal every day. We want to enlist you as a fellow caregiver to seek this standard in your own caregiving. We believe one of the best ways we can serve a patient well is to respect the vital role you play as a member of the health-care team. Our hospital's culture is a caring and compassionate one, which means we care about you and desire to shower you with kindness and appreciation as well as remind you of your important role in the life of your loved one.

One way we partner with you is to create an optimum environment for healing. A gardener knows she isn't the one causing the garden to grow. God does that. However, certain activities increase the likelihood of good growth, such as watering, fertilizing, using quality seeds, and regularly weeding. Once a gardener has done all this, the rest is up to God. Like gardeners, we health-care professionals understand our limits, but we also understand the kinds of activities that increase the probability for a successful outcome. Therefore, our "Mother Standard" requires us to do the following:

- Care about the patient as though he or she were a member of our own family. For us, there is no substitute for sincerity, and we sincerely desire wellness for every patient we see. This is our obsession.

- Explore ways of enhancing a patient's quality of life—how we can best serve him or her during this time of need. This often includes caring for the caregiver.
- Do our best to provide relief from suffering. We believe true relief comes through treating the whole person.

You are invited to share in our obsession for life—life abundant, healed, balanced, unstressed, and eternal.

If we focused our caregiving energies solely on the administration of drugs or the execution of surgical remedies, we would be irresponsible. As critical as these are to creating the optimum environment for healing, we know too much about the complexities of disease and the human condition to merely treat the condition or symptoms without addressing the underlying causes. Therefore, our treatment requires us to explore a little harder, probe a little deeper, and engage our patients at different levels of emotional and spiritual meaning to provide the quality of care that would be suitable for our own mother.

NO ONE IS CANCER FREE

Simply shrinking or removing a tumor isn't good enough for us. Why? Consider this: The average adult has between sixty and a hundred trillion cells in his or her body. Our bodies produce millions of cancer cells every day. In other words, no one is cancer free. When we speak of being cancer free, what we mean is that the cancer in our bodies hasn't formed into an identifiable tumor. This is one of the primary reasons the Cancer Treatment Centers of America believes in the importance of pastoral care and mind/body medicine.

We know that if we do not treat underlying spiritual and emotional issues, the likelihood of the immune system regaining its ability to successfully defend the body against the continual presence of cancer is less likely. We know that if we don't treat the whole person, another tumor might appear. True, it might appear anyway, but it won't be due to our neglect of the wide range of needs we know our patients are experiencing. Excellence demands more.

YOUR ATTITUDE COUNTS

Right now, the most important thing you have going for you (or against you) may be your attitude toward disease, in general, and your loved one's plight, in particular.

Ordinarily people prefer to be around others who are happy and upbeat. Although there are times when we want people to identify with our pain and empathize with our sad and difficult situations, we usually do not seek out depressed people to befriend. Why?

Because depressed people depress people! Bored people bore people! Miserable people have a way of dragging us into their world of sadness. It is true that misery loves company. We all remember times when we've been unhappy and friends came to visit us. But they didn't come to make us miserable; they came to cheer us up! To gladden our hearts. To replace our frowns with smiles. What kind of friend would we be if we left our friends more depressed than when we found them?

Caregiving is a great privilege, and it is as demanding as it is rewarding. To do it well requires us to examine our own attitudes. We need to assess our beliefs about disease and discomfort and how we face difficulties in our own lives. Why? Because your friend is depending on you, and if you fear death and cannot see the benefits of disease (the lessons our bodies are trying to teach us), you may find your capacity to care for your loved one diminished and your ability to be light during his or her period of darkness dimmed.

Caring for your loved one can be one of the most rewarding experiences of your life—a time when you experience optimum emotional, spiritual, psychological, and physical well-being, so that in return you are able to help your loved one share similar experiences.

Water cannot flow higher than its source. The source of a river or fountain is the highest geographical elevation. As gravity applies itself, the water flows from its highest elevation to its lowest. The

Mississippi River is the longest and largest river in North America. Its source is Lake Itasca in the Minnesota North Woods. It flows through the midcontinental United States, the Gulf of Mexico Coastal Plain, and its subtropical Louisiana Delta. It is all downhill from Lake Itasca.

In other words, you will not be able to raise your loved one's spirits any higher than your own spirits are raised. A positive attitude can be infectious! A strong will to live can be shared! Reasons to fight for your loved one's life can be discovered, but little or none of this will happen if the caregiver is not optimistic and otherwise happy. How can a caregiver convincingly convey the need to fight for health and longer life if he or she is indifferent and unenthused about life and living?

The Scriptures teach, "Be *joyful* always; pray continually; give thanks in all circumstances, for this is God's will for you" (1 Thess. 5:16–18).

People of faith, especially Christians, are instructed to be joyful always and are reminded that a joy-filled life is God's will. Yet joy eludes many people, especially those who are living an already busy life and are responsible for others' well-being. Ask any parent, teacher, or CEO!

Fish! is a short yet powerful book about a woman who finds herself working in a "toxic energy dump." She walks by Pike Place Fish Market, where there are a number of men working behind the counter. Suddenly she sees a fish flying through the air and hears one of the men yell out, "One salmon flying away to Minnesota!" only to be echoed just as loudly by another, "One salmon flying away to Minnesota!"[3] Soon thereafter another man tosses a coworker a bunch of crabs, yelling, "Five crabs flying away to Wisconsin!" This woman saw that the men at Pike Place Fish Market were filled with lively energy and were having a joyful time throwing fish around all day, and she began to wonder why she wasn't enjoying her job, which in her mind was much more important than selling fish. As she reflected on this, she decided her life was too precious to spend any time at all, let alone half her waking hours, in a "toxic energy dump" filled with people who were a drag to be around—unhappy and unfulfilled.

Consider the wisdom of Scripture: "A cheerful heart is good medicine, but a crushed spirit dries up the bones" (Prov. 17:22). Your friend needs good "medicine" flowing from your cheerful heart into his or hers. As Ben Franklin put it, "The Constitution only gives people the right to pursue happiness. You have to catch it yourself."[4]

Your challenge, and mine, is to create space in the life of your friend that is the emotional opposite of a toxic energy dump; one that is filled with positive energy, hope, abundant love, occasional laughter, and people engaged with life and living—people who sparkle, even in the midst of difficulty.

ELUSIVE EMOTIONS

The problem with happiness and joy is that it eludes many of us.[5] We spend a lot of time trying to figure out how to become happy. We often think money will bring us happiness, only to discover that some of the unhappiest people in the world have all the money they could ever possibly want. There is little correlation between happiness and wealth.

Some people seek happiness through social relationships, believing the answer to their problems lies in the hands of other people. And yet, relationships often suffer. A close look at married people reveals that often couples are bored to tears. Their married life is dull, drab, and gray. Why? Marriages suffer, not because the spouses do not initially love one another, but because they never learned how to remain happy.

James Allen, a nineteenth-century English author, compares our minds to gardens. Left untended, he said, they will become filled with weeds.

> A man's mind may be likened to a garden, which may be intelli-
> gently cultivated or allowed to run wild; but whether cultivated or
> neglected, it must, and will, bring forth. If no useful seeds are put

into it, then an abundance of useless weed seeds will fall therein, and will continue to produce their kind.

Just as a gardener cultivates his plot, keeping it free from weeds, and growing the flowers and fruits which he requires, so may a man tend the garden of his mind, weeding out all the wrong, useless, and impure thoughts, and cultivating toward perfection the flowers and fruits of right, useful, and pure thoughts. By pursuing this process, a man sooner or later discovers that he is the master gardener of his soul, the director of his life. He also reveals, within himself, the laws of thought, and understands with ever-increasing accuracy, how the thought forces and mind elements operate in the shaping of his character, circumstances, and destiny.[6]

Allen suggested the primary reason there are so many unhappy people is that their minds are full of weeds. This is true of human friendships as well; they must be cultivated.

For example, people enter into marriages seeking happiness, and reasonably so. No one enters into marriage anticipating failure, boredom, and frustration. The problem often lies in the unfair expectation that the spouse will be their primary source of happiness and well-being. Ultimately, if we aren't basically happy people, it's unlikely someone else can transform us into something we're not constitutionally hardwired to be. As someone once said, "Remember that a successful marriage depends on two things: (1) finding the right person and (2) being the right person."[7] This is true not only for marriages, but also for friendships. From a Christian standpoint, "being the right person" means trying to be as happy and joyful as possible.

People often limit themselves to random feelings of joy or settle for mundane living because they either don't know how to be happy or don't know how to re-create feelings of happiness once they have passed.

Here is the critical insight to experience joy and happiness: It takes effort.

It takes effort to
Read a book,
Memorize a Scripture passage,
Do a crossword puzzle,
Write a letter,
Phone a friend,
Go out to eat, or
Plan your day.

It takes no effort at all to stare at a wall or mindlessly watch television, both of which have the tendency to become a cancer patient's favorite pastimes.

As a caregiver, you have a choice to pull out the weed of unhappiness and boredom in pursuit of happiness and joy or allow the garden of your mind to become filled with weeds of despair and depression. You can make your loved one unhappy because you are unhappy. You can stress them out if you haven't developed strong coping mechanisms to deal with life's problems. But remember that God desires joy for you, even during those difficult times.

Among the many coping mechanisms that will be shared in the following chapters, let me share the one that will be echoed throughout the book as the most important one: Trust God. If you are depressed, battle your depression by trusting in God's goodness and love. Otherwise you may leave your loved one in despair. However, if you are joyful, you can teach your loved one a way of life that is superior and worth living.

You can teach them by your words, but you will be able to teach them best by your own example. As Oliver Goldsmith put it, "You can preach a better sermon with your life than with your lips."

POSITIVE PATH

Years of ministry have made me aware that people are suspicious of pastors or other religious people who appear to promote the latest in pop psychology. They distance themselves from new theories or modern attempts to understand the attitudes and beliefs that can affect human behavior.

Yet there are wonderful advancements in the field of "positive" psychology that attempt to enable individuals to experience physical and emotional blessings scientifically proven to enhance overall well-being, quality of life, cardiovascular system, and immune function. Those who question the validity of modern positive psychology may not realize it's not so modern after all. In fact, it is as old as the Scriptures themselves.

Paul wrote, "Finally, brothers, whatever is true, whatever is noble, whatever is right, whatever is pure, whatever is lovely, whatever is admirable—if anything is excellent or praiseworthy—think about such things. Whatever you have learned or received or heard from me, or seen in me—put it into practice. And the God of peace will be with you" (Phil. 4:8–9).

Without the benefit of modern scientific research, the apostle Paul knew intuitively the power of the human mind to help generate positive feelings. By encouraging his readers to focus on positive attributes or values, he was helping them to experience personal peace.

Jesus said, "Whatever you ask for in prayer, believe that you have received it, and it will be yours" (Mark 11:24). This is positive thinking put to prayer, isn't it? Modern psychology often, though not always, validates ancient biblical wisdom. For example, Jesus said, "Who of you by worrying can add a single hour to his life?" (Matt. 6:27). Implicit in this statement, it seems to me, is the belief that there might be a relationship between our worrying and the quantity of our life—millennia before research would prove the relationship between stress and immune function and cardiovascular disease. Also, secular researchers have concluded that the process of forgiveness is not complete until a person reaches the point where he or she returns to a love for or positive attitude toward the offender. They thus corroborate Jesus' instruction to his disciples to "forgive … from your heart" (Matt. 18:35).

Although positive psychology uses different methods and unfamiliar language to encourage positive feelings, it does not travel a new road, but rather finds anew an old path that can lead to an enhancement of the quality of human life. Consider this study by the Institute of HeartMath that demonstrated a link between emotion and immune function:

> Groups of volunteers were asked to focus on two different emotions—anger and care—while a key immune system antibody, secretory IgA, was being measured. IgA (immunoglobulin A) is widespread in the immune system, acting as a protective coating for the cells against invading bacteria or viruses. Stress is known to decrease IgA levels, leaving us more vulnerable to respiratory problems such as colds or flus. The study found that a five-minute period of recalling an angry experience caused a six-hour suppression of IgA levels. Five minutes of sincerely feeling care or compassion, on the other hand, boosted IgA levels for six hours.[8]

Knowing this, don't you feel compelled to help your loved one experience compassion? I know I do.

DISCOVER A BETTER WAY

Are you sad and dejected? Are you overwrought with distress? Are you overwhelmed with worry and concern? Are you angry? Emotionally exhausted? Bored?

These understandable emotions probably reflect the attitude of many, if not most, cancer patients and caregivers. After all, a life-threatening disease or chronic illness isn't something we would wish on anyone. We spend much time and energy trying to avoid being sick. We dress warmly when it's cold. We avoid being around people who are coughing and sneezing. We make late-night trips to the drugstore to pick up prescription or over-the-counter drugs that will make us feel better or sleep well. Surely, no one wants to be sick. No one desires to suffer.

Boredom, exhaustion, anger, worry, and feeling miserable are how many people choose to "do" life. When people are faced with chronic or life-threatening disease, all of these emotions are understandable. But they aren't necessary, helpful, or productive in your life or in the life of your friend.

Now is the time for you to discover—if you haven't already—how to live! You and your friend can learn some of the great lessons other people have discovered during the difficult moments in their lives.

Consider the apostle Paul. He wrote some of his most beautiful letters while he was under house arrest in a Roman jail. The following describes his attitude: "Everything happening to me in this jail only serves to make Christ more accurately known, regardless of whether I live or die. They didn't shut me up; they gave me a pulpit! Alive, I'm Christ's messenger; dead, I'm his bounty. Life versus even more life! I can't lose" (Phil. 1:20–21 MSG).

Paul was stuck. Going nowhere. Facing the possibility that his life might end. The only pleasures he enjoyed were his friends—Timothy and Epaphroditus—and writing letters to the churches he founded. And yet he was able to look at his life through a very special lens: one filled with hope, optimism, and joy. How? He had an attitude that would not allow him to succumb to despair. In spite of his unknown future, in conditions that must have been less than desirable, he wrote these words:

> Summing it all up, friends, I'd say you'll do best by filling your
> minds and meditating on things true, noble, reputable, authentic,
> compelling, gracious—the best, not the worst; the beautiful, not the
> ugly; things to praise, not things to curse. Put into practice what you
> learned from me, what you heard and saw and realized. Do that,
> and God, who makes everything work together, will work you into
> his most excellent harmonies. (Phil. 4:8–9 MSG)

With many reasons to be sad, downhearted, and ill-tempered, Paul was a beacon of optimism, hope, and joy. How did he manage that? Do you wonder if you could too? Perhaps you feel stuck, struggling with helping someone whom you may not even want to help, wishing someone else would engage in the caregiving.

Being stuck is a state of mind. It is something you choose to embrace or reject. As I will discuss later, being stuck may simply be the result of poor pastime management.

DEVELOP A HIGH "GET IT" FACTOR

One of the most marvelous experiences I have had as a professional caregiver is witnessing cancer patients who, over time, develop what I call a high "get it" factor. These are people who have embraced the following realities:

- Life is short—for everyone. Therefore, now is the time to gently and slowly make whatever adjustments are needed to move into equilibrium—spiritually, emotionally, and physically.
- Union with God is impossible without loving and forgiving others as well as ourselves.
- Our bodies are wonderful gifts from a good and gracious God. Taking care of our bodies through exercise and eating well can be a joyful endeavor, even a spiritual one.
- The best defense against the ravaging effects of aging, in general, or cancer, in particular, is living a well-balanced life wherein our immune system operates optimally.
- Social support from friends and family is a critical component to the healing equation.
- Worrying about tomorrow is less productive than living a happy, fulfilled life today. Today is to be treasured and not taken for granted.
- Joy and happiness are not acquired by those who are able to remove all problems from their life, but rather by those who respond to life's problems with optimism and hope—an inner attitude grounded in a belief in a big God who makes all hurdles small.

- Life is a game we cannot win but can learn to enjoy. Make a game out of every day.
- Trusting God is more than a cliché, it is a lifestyle. It's important to trust God with every moment of every day, not just with what happens when we die.

People who have a high "get it" factor have an unwavering trust in God. Their faith is joyful, humble, and often infectious. It is as though they live by rules most people either do not understand or only experience on a handful of occasions during their lifetime. These people seem to be walking on clouds even though they have their feet firmly planted in reality.

My goal—and yours—as a caregiver is to introduce patients to living in hope so they can truly experience this vibrant life. Not for tomorrow—because none of us knows what tomorrow will bring—but for today. This is a lot easier said than done, but it is particularly important for those who face life-threatening disease.

Which would you prefer: ten years of living miserably or hope-filled joy today? I know I would prefer to have joy today and to leave the uncertain future to God. By bringing your loved one's life into balance, his or her immune system will function at its highest level, giving him or her the best chance of overcoming cancer's ravaging effects.

HOPE OR PITY?

All too often we treat people who are suffering with sadness and pity. And while sympathy and sadness are sometimes appropriate, I wouldn't want to be continually surrounded by morose, depressed, and gloomy people, would you? Compassionate caregiving isn't merely cutting out tumors, administering chemotherapy, or even anointing with oil and offering prayer. Compassionate caregiving also requires lifting a person's spirits!

In the end, all we have to offer people who experience broken-ness in life, whether the brokenness is cancer, HIV/AIDS, limb amputation, divorce, or a stubbed toe, is pity or hope. We can either feel sorry for them, or we can offer them a future filled with wonderful possibilities, including hope for restoration and new beginnings, by helping them realize the best route to a wonderful tomorrow is a joyful, though not always painless, today.

The Scriptures teach about a God who "redeems [our] life from the pit," who satisfies our desires with "good things" so that our "youth is renewed like the eagle's" (Ps. 103:4–5). How does God do this? He does it by sending people into our lives who lift our spirits, make us smile, care about the condition of our hearts and souls, and make us feel young again.

As God cares for us, we ought also to care for others. Primary care can be about life and living or death and dying—it can be a continuation of the Spirit's display of love and joy.[9]

Chapter Two

Principles of Caregiving

All artists use tools of one kind or another. Whether it is a paintbrush or a scalpel, a hammer or a lug wrench, everyone has his or her own tools of the trade. Caregiving is no less an art with its own unique set of tools, the most important being wisdom.

To be sure, having the desire or heartfelt commitment to care for a loved one is a great tool or weapon against despair, pain, and a wavering faith. As they say in the South, "You gotta wanna." However, having the desire to help someone in need, regardless of whether that need is lung cancer or a sore throat, isn't enough. For example, wanting to be a good parent is admirable, but if the person doesn't have any parenting skills he or she may end up doing as much harm to the child as good. Good caregiving, like good parenting, improves greatly from learning a few tools of the trade.

I have compiled a list of significant caregiving tools, or principles, I use daily in my pastoral care to cancer patients, tools that help me keep my sanity while helping others. I call them "heart lessons." Knowing these lessons, I believe, will enhance the quality of your caregiving experience and create a wonderful environment for good things to happen to you as well as to the one you are committed to caring for. With God's help, these heart lessons should make caregiving, as difficult as it can be at times, a meaningful and joyful experience.

Heart Lesson 1: The Unordained Caregiver

The doctors told him that if he didn't have coronary bypass surgery soon he would die.

He refused the surgery. Repeatedly.

As a seminarian, part of my theological training included participating in a summerlong hospital chaplaincy program. One of my
greatest disappointments that summer was my inability to convince
this forty-five-year-old man that he ought to have bypass surgery. I
talked with him. I prayed with him. I pulled every rabbit out of my
theological hat in order to convince him that life was good and well
worth living. He responded that he was unemployed and divorced
and couldn't think of one reason to want to live.

Dejected, I spoke with my supervisor about the situation, and he
said, "Mike, you know what the problem is, don't you?"

"No."

"He hasn't ordained you to be his pastor. His fishing buddy could
have him on the operating table in ten minutes!"

I've never forgotten that lesson. I did not have a deep enough
friendship with this man to inspire him to do what he needed to do to
live. His closest friend could and mostly likely would have that kind of
not-so-subtle influence over him. Such is the power and potential
influence a close friend can have at critical moments in our lives. You,
as a caregiver, may have as much or more influence in the life of your
loved one than anyone on the health-care team.

Mark Twain once said, "The difference between the almost right
word and the right word is really a large matter—it's the difference
between the lightning bug and the lightning."[1] If you have your
friend's fishing-buddy trust, you have the opportunity to speak the
right word—a word that has the effect of lightning in his or her life.
Please be aware of the tremendous influence you have, and do not
keep "lightning" to yourself. You may be the only person on the
health-care team who can speak the right word at the right time.

However, fishing-buddy trust can never be assumed by a caregiver.
One afternoon I saw a husband and wife sitting in the cafeteria. I knew
them, having had several brief conversations with them in the past.
The wife was very frustrated by her husband's unwillingness to accept
a treatment plan that made sense to her and their oncologist. Sensing

the possibility that the wife might not be his "ordained" caregiver, I gently shared some stories about my experiences with caregiving, times when I felt ineffective and unordained. Not surprisingly, the wife matter-of-factly declared she was not her husband's ordained caregiver, a statement he didn't argue with or contradict.

I knew bringing this subject up was potentially risky, but it seemed the right moment to help them understand how and why they had reached a stalemate in their discussion about future care. Further, I hoped I might be able to help them learn how to build a bridge back into each other's world.

Ordination issues are very real, and they are as unspoken as they are common. The human heart is complex. No one knows how or why people fall in or out of love. They just do. No one can predict the tipping point between friendship and love, love and hatred, trust and distrust. One moment you are friends, and the next moment your feelings are different, and so it goes. The sparkle of romance is often altered by the daily routine of life, and years of hard work and child rearing can cause even the most devoted relationships and the deepest feelings of love to lose their luster. Human beings are often contrary and unpredictable—and yet still worth loving, redeeming, and caring for, their contrariness notwithstanding.

My wife's elderly mother needed full-time care. My wife convinced her to move out of her home into a health-care facility. Shortly after she established her new residence, my mother-in-law began to miss home and longed to return. As her complaining reached fever pitch, my wife was forced to travel thousands of miles to try to convince her it was in her best interest to stay where she was. But my wife, my wife's sister, and her aunt did not appear to be ordained by my mother-in-law to convince her to stay. Who was? The family halfheartedly confessed it was a little old lady named Rita she'd befriended at a local cafeteria, someone my wife and family had never even met! In sum, a virtual stranger was the "chosen one."

As I described this psychosocial "Rita" phenomenon to a cancer support group at Willow Creek Community Church in South

Barrington, Illinois, one of the attendees yelled out, "No! Her name isn't Rita! It's Lois!" She told of her own experience, and we all had a good laugh, albeit a nervous and somewhat painful one.

Is it hurtful to be passed over in this type of situation? Yes, of course, but there is nothing that can quickly change relationships that have evolved over many, many decades. They are what they are.

My reason for explaining this psychosocial phenomenon is three-fold: to prepare you for the possibility of this kind of disappointment, to help you think about whom you might be able to bring into the decision-making process to facilitate adequate care, and to be aware that you—and you alone—may be the only ordained caregiver on the health-care team!

Moving from being "unordained" to "ordained" is a challenge every therapist, pastor, chaplain, and counselor regularly faces. Daily, professional therapists work with clients who are highly unmotivated to be there with them. Often a client feels forced into the therapeutic relationship by a parent, a spouse, the judicial system, and so forth. Therapists know they are not automatically ordained to help their client and that learning how to respond to this challenge requires skillful training and a great deal of patience and experience.

It is possible to gain or regain a loved one's total trust—fishing-buddy trust—but many of us do not have the skills or time it takes. Because of this, it's healthy to accept the possibility that in spite of your enormous love and effort, when it comes to making critical decisions about your loved one's care, your advice may not be sought or taken seriously. Please resist the temptation to get angry and defensive. In the end, what is most important is your loved one's health, not your feelings.

HEART LESSON 2: YOU CANNOT MOTIVATE THE UNMOTIVATED

Another important lesson for all caregivers to learn is that *you cannot give insights to unmotivated people.* For me as a pastor who has preached virtually every Sunday morning for more than fifteen years, this lesson has been invaluable in helping me maintain my sanity. It reminds me that the words of the best preacher in the world are useless unless the listeners are motivated to listen. Put another way, if his or her students do not want to learn, it doesn't matter how gifted or talented the teacher may be.

In his book *Friedman's Fables*, the late psychologist Edwin Friedman makes this point with a humorous story about a man who desires to teach his wife how to play tennis. He buys her the best equipment and a lovely tennis outfit, carefully positions her on the tennis court, and offers instruction on how to hit the ball when it comes to her. Then he runs to the other side of the net and softly hits a ball toward her. The ball bounces right by her, and she doesn't move a muscle. The husband returns to his wife and rehearses the movement with similar results. After going through this routine five times, he finally hits the ball very high in the air across the net and runs around to the other side where he hits it back to himself. The moral of the story: His wife didn't want to learn to play tennis![2] Remember, you cannot give insights to unmotivated people!

This is a hard lesson when the stakes are much higher than learning to play a game of tennis. What do we do when loved ones don't want to live? When they refuse to fight for their life? What do we do when they won't eat or exercise properly? When they continually fill their minds with negative self-talk?

A caregiver's power to force anyone to do anything is limited. We can nag, push, cajole, yell, scream, demand, and beg, but the bottom line is this: If your loved one isn't motivated to do what you want him or her to do, your energy will be wasted, along with your hopes and dreams. Of course, my hope and prayer is that your loved one will be motivated to listen and learn from you. In the end, though, only God can soften a hardened heart. Be patient and pray.

HEART LESSON 3: CHANGE TAKES TIME

Cancer treatment is often a slow process—snail-like slow. I work at a hospital that streamlines procedures for maximum effectiveness and, due to "lean" thinking, has been successful in its attempts to remove barriers to speedy treatment. Yet from the patient's point of view, everything often still seems to take forever. If ever there was a time for patience, now is that time. The changes that need to take place physically will take time. Changes in the spiritual and emotional worlds take time too. For example, many people with cancer have experienced deep spiritual wounds that can only be healed by forgiveness. Forgiveness is a process that takes time. Learning to trust God takes time—sometimes a long time. It takes time to quit smoking. It takes time to develop healthier eating habits. It takes time to learn to better manage our emotions.

Most Christians are frequently challenged by the apostle Paul's advice to be "transformed by the renewing of [our] mind[s]" (Rom. 12:2). But how, exactly, are our minds "transformed"? Because of the importance of thinking optimistically, how can I as a caregiver help cancer patients make necessary changes in their thought processes and lifestyle? Change is possible, but it often takes time. Of all the important changes a person might need to make, the change that is the easiest, and perhaps the most beneficial from a quality of life standpoint, is the decision to choose to do things that bring happiness.

Of my many bits of advice I give to cancer patients and their caregivers, few are repeated more than this: Today is the only day we know for certain that we are going to be alive. No one knows if he or she will be alive tomorrow. All we have is today. Twenty-four hours. We can choose to fill our time doing things that bring us some sense of happiness and joy, or we can spend it being depressed, unhappy, and pessimistic. Choose to fill your time doing things that bring you some measure of happiness and peace, even if it is as simple as listening to music you love. Or you can sit around the waiting room staring at the walls or lie in bed feeling sorry for yourself. Twenty-four hours. How are you going to spend it? Being happy or sad? You choose.

HEART LESSON 4: PUSH GENTLY, BUT PUSH!

Ordinarily I would caution caregivers not to push (strongly encourage) loved ones to do something they may or may not want to do. Perhaps you have heard of the law of inverse proportion. If you have a child (especially a teenager), you have seen this law in action many times: the harder you push, the greater the resistance. Yet unlike your children, your hurting friend may have very little time to live—pushing may be not only your best course of action, but also the only hope.

Recent research suggests that many cancer patients suffer from "chronic niceness." They are so nice that they allow people to walk all over them. And when this happens, they often become angry and turn that anger inward, which eats away at them and may even contribute to their developing cancer.

Chronic niceness makes many patients passive. This passivity can even affect their health care.

One problem is that some hospitals and medical professionals act as though they are doing patients a favor by helping them. The hubris exhibited is shocking.

For instance, a cancer patient and her husband told me about their oncologist's behavior after informing them that, in his opinion, there was no more hope for them; they should go home and get their affairs in order. Tearfully, the woman with cancer asked if there wasn't anything that could be done for her—she refused to give up. She said the doctor angrily threw his pen on his desk and walked out of his office.

One gentleman told me the only reason he was at a new hospital was because of his wife's heroic efforts. She made the phone calls to the cancer hospital. She arranged to have the medical records sent from the oncologist to the new cancer-care provider. Her assertiveness may have saved her husband's life. She was pushy because her options were limited and time was growing short. When our loved ones are too passive about their own health outcomes, sometimes more aggressive measures are required. Occasionally I see patients who have been brought to the hospital by loving caregivers and who appear to be completely disinterested in being healed; they're almost suicidal. One such patient was a young man of thirty-five, who had been brought to the hospital by his mother. Otherwise healthy, if he would be willing to get the needed chemotherapy, he had every reason to believe he could become a long-term survivor of his disease. I was summoned to the examination room by a colleague for help. His mother was sobbing, pleading with her son to have the chemotherapy. It was heart-breaking. Such love his mother had for him. His reply? "Mother, this is my life, not yours." It took several days, but she prevailed upon him to get treatment. Sadly, he punished his mother by refusing to allow her to accompany him to the hospital while he got it.

Having said that, remember Heart Lesson 2: You cannot motivate the unmotivated. Pushing may be the only hope your loved one has and may be the only way they get checked in to a new hospital, but that doesn't mean he or she will appreciate your efforts or even coop-erate with the new medical team. For the sake of love and life, though, sometimes all we can do is push. So firmly push—and fervently pray.

My own dear mother is an example of this hard reality. She was a very beautiful woman, even at the age of sixty-seven, when she learned she had breast cancer. Following a mastectomy, she refused chemotherapy, opting for only alternative medical treatments prima-rily focused upon nutrition. She died two years later. If I only knew then what I know now, perhaps I might have been able to convince her otherwise, but she was as stubborn as she was beautiful.

Occasionally it is not just the patient who needs pushing. Sometimes health-care professionals need a nudge. Truth be known, patients are not always being served well, and they often feel power-less to move things along more quickly. At times like that, I often ask the patient or caregiver to put complaints in writing, and I promise to deliver them to the president of the hospital. We cannot always right every wrong, but we do care about all patients and their experience at our hospital.

HEART LESSON 5: HAPPINESS IS A CHOICE

Happiness and joy are choices we can make, and many people do choose to find life enjoyable even when facing life-threatening diseases or catastrophic circumstances. Scholars Martha H. Pieper, PhD, and William J. Pieper, MD, believe some people, and perhaps many, are addicted to unhappiness. In their book *Addicted to Unhappiness* they wrote,

> Our most important message is that you are never too old and it is never too late to recover from an addiction to unhappiness and embark on a life of positive, satisfying, and effective choices. The spark of inborn joy and optimism that you possessed when you entered into the world ... can be fanned into a guiding light by thoughtful, careful life planning.... Even when you are faced with the most unfortunate of events, you can learn to maintain your inner equilibrium and to avoid ... turning on yourself or others.[3]

The Bible teaches, "Choose for yourselves this day whom you will serve.... But as for me and my household, we will serve the LORD" (Josh. 24:15). The capacity to make choices is one of the primary distinctions between humans and other lower forms of existence. Happy people make life-giving choices. Not only during the good times; anyone can do that. It takes a special ability and desire to decide to be happy and joyful when times aren't so good. Choice is what connects us to God and allows us to work together with him to subdue the creation he has placed in our charge (see 2 Cor. 6:1). Without it, morality (the ability to do right or wrong) would be meaningless. Evil, due to our sin nature, would be unavoidable.

The primary choice happy people make that unhappy people do not is to shift their focus or attention from the negative to the positive. Happy people look to the good, expecting all things to work together for good (Rom. 8:28). Not some things, occasionally. But all things, always. Happy people know there is a silver lining in every dark cloud and that there are lessons to be learned and wisdom to be gained from every circumstance, especially those that threaten to break your heart or even your existence. As Dr. Dan

Baker, founder of Canyon Ranch, a popular health resort in Arizona, put it so well, "The greater the pain, the more profound the lesson."[4]

Happy people embrace pain and disappointment in anticipation of the lessons they will learn from them. They trust in a loving God and seek to find the good in their situation.

When you shift your attention toward that which is good, kind, and loving, you are making the most important first step in a journey toward happiness.

Dr. Dan Baker and Cameron Stauth conclude their book on happiness by telling a story about a woman named Emily who had cancer. Imagine ending a book on happiness with a story about a woman battling cancer! He asked her if she had learned the meaning of life.

> "The meaning of life?" She looked dead serious. "Of course I've learned the meaning of life." She smiled. "The meaning of life is to live. I think I know the secret to happiness. It's this: Every moment that has ever been, or ever will be, is gone the instant that it began. So life is loss. And the secret of happiness is to learn to love the moment more than you mourn the loss."[5]

Emily made the choice to seek happiness even as she faced cancer. She chose not to allow it to break her spirit—not to become overwhelmed with fear of death and dying. She turned a deaf ear to fear even when it screamed for attention. And so can you, if you choose to focus on God and all that is good, kind, and beautiful in the world.

HEART LESSON 6: CANCER IS A GIFT

Those of us in the caregiving field know the value of having a solid knowledge base as we prepare to offer care. It's important to understand the disease and how we, as caregivers, can best reach out to those we love. In this book, I'll answer questions like these:

What does my friend need from me right now? How can I help the most? When will I know if I am being unhelpful? What do I do if I feel like my friend isn't getting the care and support I believe is needed?

But I will also focus on other important questions, such as, How can I make the difficult task of caring for a chronically ill person a life-giving, rewarding experience? How do I return day after day to a difficult situation with an upbeat and positive attitude?

You see, I am concerned about you. Granted, I'm concerned about the quality of care you give to your friend, but I believe that it is only partially determined by the knowledge you have about the disease. The quality of the care you give is largely determined by the quality of life *you* are living and encouraging your loved one to live. Consider John Steinbeck's words: "A sad soul can kill you quicker than a germ."[6]

Now make this your caregiver prayer:

Dear God: If my friend is going to perish from a sad soul, please do not let him catch the germ from me. Amen.

What if I told you your experience as a caregiver could be life giving instead of life depleting? An experience that allows you to thrive (emotionally, spiritually, psychologically, and physically) instead of merely survive? A season of life in which sitting by your struggling friend does not fill you with dread?

What if you could learn how to experience optimum energy and capacity to enjoy life? What if you were able to view cancer as a friend willing to teach you important life lessons? Cancer does not have to be viewed as a monster.

Cancer can be viewed as a friend.

A wake-up call to a new way of living.

A spiritual revival.

One of the best things that ever happened to you and your loved one.

A gift.

Impossible? If you think so, I wonder why. If, indeed, "with God all things are possible" (Matt. 19:26), how is it that you are suspicious of the possibility that cancer might become your teacher and friend?

I know you may not be ready to hear this, but just consider the possibility that cancer can be a friend—or an enemy that has been befriended. In either event, whether we consider cancer as an enemy or a friend, remember these wise words from Antisthenes, a Greek philosopher and disciple of Socrates: "There are only two people who can tell you the truth about yourself—an enemy who has lost his temper and a friend who loves you dearly."

CHAPTER THREE

The Mental Laws of Transformation

In his book *Maximum Achievement*,[1] author Brian Tracy provides helpful advice I use every day with my cancer patients. As a caregiver, you too might find some of his "mental laws" helpful. And while exploring ways to help your loved one experience mental transformation, perhaps you'll find that your mind also becomes transformed for the better.

THE MENTAL LAW OF PRACTICE

The Mental Law of Practice suggests that our minds can be changed, resulting in new, desirable behavior. This is done by continually considering qualities and traits we want to acquire. Tracy wrote, "The Law of Practice states that whatever thought or action you repeat often enough becomes a new habit.... This is how you become a new and better person."[2]

Let me give you an example. When I was young I read the timeless classic *The Little Engine That Could*. The little engine, faced with an uphill climb that seemed insurmountable, repeatedly said to himself, "I think I can, I think I can, I think I can," which we all know resulted in his getting to the top of the hill. In reading that story, I developed a can-do attitude. Later in life, when I was faced with situations or circumstances that appeared impossible, subconsciously the Mental Law of Practice kicked in, and I began to program my mind into believing that if I applied myself I could achieve the goal I desired.

THE MENTAL LAW OF REPETITION

As Peter McWilliams once said, "A successfully communicated thought, from one human mind to another, is one of the most powerful forces I know."[3] And there is perhaps no thought more powerful or important to communicate than the *power* of such a positive thought continually repeated until it sinks into our heads and then into our hearts, where a new reality is created. Our minds can be transformed, but it takes both repetition and patience.

For example, I have never had a patient or parishioner come to me after a sermon and say, "That sermon just changed my life!" Often, though, people take the thoughts I've shared with them home, where they either consciously or unconsciously ponder them. After having chewed this information, occasionally they find themselves in the grip of a new reality. The Word can sink into the mind quickly, but often the heart digests it slowly.

The story of my patient C.P. is a good illustration of the power of a pondered thought. Part of my role as a chaplain is to communicate the importance of faith in the healing equation, that the condition of our soul often has an effect on the wellness of our body. Because forgiveness is often an issue with patients, I frequently use it to illustrate the relationship between faith and health.

C.P. came into my office one afternoon burdened by her past. She wrote in her testimonial, "The most important thing I seemed to keep avoiding was trying to get my spiritual connection in tune with my body." Like many, she had not thought much about faith issues, much less the importance of forgiveness in a Christian's life. Again, she wrote,

> At three a.m. I decided to begin to pray.... As I lay there begging God for some peace to sleep, I began to feel a warmth come over me, a warmth of peace that I had never experienced before. I soon realized that I was in the presence of God. The first revelation he revealed to me was that the reason Jesus came to earth was to forgive us of our sins. But he also revealed to me that people need

to forgive [others] because without true forgiveness, it blocks the channel to where our souls can communicate with God.

God enabled her to forgive someone who had hurt her deeply. "I have now forgiven, and yes, love the souls I forgave without any hesitation or resistance. What a beautiful divine feeling to have!" She learned that her unforgiveness had become a "hindrance to her journey with God." As she continually pondered God, her faith, and forgiveness, he transformed her mind. In God's timing, he met her at her point of need.

Repeating good thoughts is as powerful as it is simple. The Mental Law of Repetition teaches us that continual exposure to positive thoughts produces positive outcomes—a healthier soul if not a cured body. All caregivers ought to bathe their minds in good thoughts, and to the best of their ability encourage their loved ones to do the same. Good thoughts are always candlelight to the soul.

As I will address more fully later, it is very difficult for cancer patients to concentrate on anything for any length of time; such is their mental condition. Thoughts and feelings are often moving targets. Help your loved one focus on one positive thought as a way to anchor his or her mind in goodness. For example, have the person repeat, "With God's help, I'm going to be healed"; or "With God all things are possible" (Matt. 19:26); or perhaps the best verse to ponder is "Not my will, but yours be done" (Luke 22:42)—anything that allows him or her to concentrate on positive outcomes or peaceful states of being. But be cautious.

Many faithful Christians claim that by simply believing they are healed of cancer (or speaking those words aloud) it will be so. Here is the reality I face as a chaplain in a cancer hospital: Everyone reading this book will be dead in less than a hundred years. Even the most devout and faithful. I know Scripture teaches us that "whatever you ask for in prayer, believe that you have received it, and it will be yours" (Mark 11:24). Nevertheless I have lost many a patient and friend to cancer, their faith and prayers notwithstanding. Like you, I am left to ponder the meaning of this verse, but I am never left with hopelessness and despair. Rather, as I place my faith in a God who did not spare his Son, I can only conclude that this was their appointed time to return to the Father.

The key here is to encourage your loved one to repeat the positive thought or phrase over and over again. It will serve as a spiritual anchor in a sea of mindless chaos; it will help steady the person spiritually for whatever he or she may face next.

As Samuel Johnson once wrote,

> All the performances of human art, at which we look with praise or wonder, are instances of the resistless force of perseverance; it is by this that the quarry becomes a pyramid, and that distant countries are united with canals. If a man was to compare the single stroke of the pickaxe, or of one impression of the spade, with the general design and the last result, he would be overwhelmed by the sense of their disproportion; yet those petty operations, incessantly continued, in time surmount the greatest difficulties, and mountains are leveled and oceans bounded by the slender force of human beings.[4]

I believe positive, good, holy thoughts and prayers are each a "stroke of the pickaxe" that lead to an experience of the "God of peace" (Phil. 4:9).

THE MENTAL LAW OF RELAXATION

Another one of Tracy's laws, one that complements the Laws of Practice and Repetition, is the Mental Law of Relaxation. This law suggests that change is accomplished differently in the mental world than it is in the physical. He offers as an illustration the experience of cutting a log in half. In the physical world, hard work and a sharp ax will help the cutter achieve quick success. However, the opposite is true in the spiritual and emotional worlds: Hard work is often counterproductive. It can often create internal crisis, stress, and guilt, inhibiting the likelihood of positive outcome. Granted, crises and godly guilt often precede spiritual renewal and regeneration. However, when a patient's immune system is already severely compromised, I believe there are more loving ways to accomplish the same purpose of renewal. As the Scriptures teach us, "'Not by might nor by power, but by my Spirit,' says the LORD Almighty" (Zech. 4:6). Trust the Spirit of God to gently work in the life of your loved one.

This is an important law to understand, particularly for you as a caregiver. If I were to teach patients about a correlation between faith and health, some might respond, "Oh no, I don't have enough faith! I'd better start reading my Bible more, going to church more regularly!" and so forth. This kind of "work harder" thinking can cause fear, anxiety, worry, and stress, which is the opposite of the peace God wants his people to enjoy. Regular church attendance and daily Bible reading are good habits to develop, but the desired change or sought-after benefits of faith may take time to cultivate.

Positive change occurs only when we allow our minds to sit gently with a new idea or new thought. Sit calmly and confidently with a desirable outcome in mind, and trust that over time it will come to pass. Plant the seeds of positive thoughts, and allow God to water and nurture them and bring them through the crusty earth into reality.

The apostle Paul encouraged his beloved church in Philippi to think on whatever is true, noble, right, pure, lovely, admirable, excellent, and praiseworthy (Phil. 4:8). What might the outcome be if we gently and confidently pondered these words and the desirable virtues they represent?

Gently pondering *truth* will, over time, make us more uncomfortable with anything that is false.

Gently pondering *nobility* will, over time, help us gain a sense of confidence that we will be able to defeat whatever dragons we will encounter on the road ahead.

Gently pondering that which is *right* helps us gain confidence that although we are not always right, God's grace is sufficient for us.

Gently pondering *purity* reminds us that those who are "pure in heart ... will see God" (Matt. 5:8). Over time, pondering purity will help us to better see God at work in our own life as well as in the lives of those around us.

Gently pondering that which is *lovely* will, over time, allow us to see the beauty that is in the world.

Gently pondering that which is *admirable* will, over time, lead us to admire others while helping shape how others see us.

Gently pondering *excellence* will, over time, cause us to resist the temptation to settle for mediocrity.

Gently pondering that which is *worthy of praise* will, over time, lead us back to the source of all that is good, lovely, and worthy of praise: God himself.

Gently ponder this thought: "O LORD my God, I called to you for help and you healed me" (Ps. 30:2).

As you and your loved one confidently, yet gently, ponder this thought, in time your souls will respond positively and along with them, your bodies.

THE MENTAL LAW OF BELIEF WITH FEELING

The Mental Law of Belief with Feeling teaches us that slowly but surely our minds are capable of creating a new reality for us, but only if we are passionate about accomplishing the goals we desire. Harvard Medical School teaches its medical students, "What you believe is what you become." The Scriptures share similar wisdom: "As he thinketh in his heart, so is he" (Prov. 23:7 KJV). These teachings presume a passionate desire to achieve goals.

I passionately believe that the life of every patient is precious and that I can help effect a better health outcome for my patients if they are willing to cooperate.

Here's an example of what I mean. A wonderful man in my former congregation learned he had a late-stage form of an aggressive cancer. At that stage, the statistics suggest that only 1 to 3 percent of patients will be alive in thirty months. That's a mere two-and-a-half

years, and most people live only a few months. As I entered this man's
life, I prayed with him and taught him about the importance of living
for the day, being grateful for his daily bread, loving his wife, spoiling
his children and grandchildren, playing golf, and having fun without
worrying about his cancer. I filled him, as best I could, with the
candlelight of encouragement, optimism, and faith in God. I helped
him to believe that, as the philosopher Cicero once said, "While
there's life, there's hope."[5]

He not only beat the odds of living two-and-a-half years, he
almost doubled it! I believed with God-inspired passion that his life
could be dramatically extended if he would cooperate with my trying
to help him. Although he did not overcome his disease, his body
responded positively because he came to believe it too.

I am not encouraging you to put your faith in faith. I am encouraging you to put your faith in God, believing that your friend can live
longer, with a higher level of quality, if he or she believes that with
God anything is possible. But don't forget, you're not going to be able
to convince your loved one of it if you are not convinced of it yourself.

THE MENTAL LAW OF CONFIDENT EXPECTATION

The Mental Law of Confident Expectation is often referred to as
the self-fulfilling prophecy. Tracy suggests that if we confidently
expect positive results, they will, over time, come to pass. The opposite is also true—if we do not expect good things to happen, they
probably won't.

This law ought to be inscribed on the wall of every medical school
in the country. If medical professionals better understood the power
of the mind to effect positive outcomes, well-meaning doctors
wouldn't have to default to telling their patients "there is no hope" or
"this would be a good time to get your affairs in order." Christians are
taught to always have their affairs in order. We understand that we are
to always live in watchful anticipation of our unexpected return to the
Father (Luke 12:40). Nevertheless, it is one thing to tell patients that
there is nothing more that *you* (the doctor) can do for them, and

quite another to tell them that there is nothing at all that can be done. Again, I am not naive. Many of my patients have left the hospital to return to their homes to die under the compassionate care of their local hospice organization. On the other hand, their diagnosis might be medical hubris.

Although it may seem true that the likelihood of recovery is minimal, in fact it may not be true at all! But once doctors use their power to suggest a confident expectation of death, have they all but signed their patient's death certificate? Perhaps, especially *if the patient believes them.*

I can tell you story after story of patients who chose not to believe their doctors' diagnoses and are alive today—often decades later—because they had a confident expectation they were going to beat the disease.

Tracy offers a helpful metaphor to illustrate this point: Confident expectations are life's "coming attractions." Anyone who has been to a movie knows what it's like to watch five or six movie trailers before the main feature begins. Like these movie trailers, life's coming attractions are right now being shown on the silver screen of your mind! Whatever you confidently expect and believe is "coming soon" in your life will likely play itself out in your future.

How does that relate to your role as caregiver? If you and your loved one don't confidently believe in the possibility of healing, it will be much more difficult for the medical team to bring you both to that hopeful reality. To be sure, there may be underlying reasons causing you to doubt that your loved one might become a long-term cancer survivor. A common reason for skepticism is that some cancer patients have had family members who have died from cancer. It is important to remember that very few known cancers are genetically based. If there is a connection, it may have more to do with nutrition and/or other learned behaviors, such as exercise or the way our bio-families learned to cope with their problems through substance abuse, whether through legal substances (food and alcohol) or illegal substances.

Stop for a moment and digest this thought: According to a study by Dr. Stephen Locke from Harvard Medical School, people with high coping mechanisms have bodies that produce three times the number of natural killer cells (NK cells are the immune system's foot soldiers in the fight against cancer) than those with low coping mechanisms. Our faith in God's love and sovereignty is our primary coping mechanism; it is, or should be, the source of our peace and relief from our immune-suppressing stress. I understand your caution and concern and even your doubts. However, if we do not draw upon the reality of God's love and mercy, we do so at our own peril.[6]

THE MENTAL LAW OF CONCENTRATION

The Mental Law of Concentration suggests that no one can concentrate on two things at one time. Keep in mind that multitasking doesn't mean we concentrate on many things at once, but rather that we're able to efficiently redirect our concentration to accomplish a wide range of tasks.

Without concentration, it is impossible to accomplish much at all. I will discuss later how life-threatening diseases can inhibit a person's capacity to concentrate. But for now, let's digest the Law of Concentration.

Our minds are like gardens. Left unattended, weeds will grow—automatically. Weeds do not need encouragement, water, nutrition, or unsurprisingly, even weeding. Tracy suggests that without intentional cultivation and the planting of flowers, our minds become filled with the weeds of negativity, worry, anxiety, and self-loathing. He suggests the reason many people are unhappy is because their minds are filled with weeds. We must plant flowers instead.

I know a young woman who suffers from self-esteem issues. She is constantly thinking self-deprecating thoughts. In essence, she is mentally abusing herself. If I did that to her or anyone else I'd probably be arrested, but she continues to do it to herself. Her mental weeds have grown so thick that the landscape of her mind is dark and negative. She is not only missing the world's beauty, but also her own.

"Plant flowers," I tell her. "When you look in the mirror, tell your-self you are pretty and talented and powerful and capable of extraor-dinary achievement!"

As your loved one's caregiver, your job is to plant flowers in his or her mind. But first, you need to plant them in your own. Let me plant one for you: You are a wonderfully courageous person who is daring to help a good friend. The world needs more people like you!

CHAPTER FOUR

Believing in Great Possibilities

---◆---

A MIND ONCE STRETCHED BY A NEW IDEA NEVER RETURNS
TO ITS ORIGINAL DIMENSIONS.

—Oliver Wendell Holmes

Consider these words from a young woman, Barbara, who is battling cancer: "Cancer has been a gift. It has made me realize what is so great about living. It has inspired me to teach my children what the important things are. No more worry. Or bad eating habits. Or anger. A year before I found out that I had cancer, my heart was broken and I *wanted* to die. These signals my body felt on the cellular level. I had to forgive."

Barbara's comments are not unusual. *Many cancer patients have told me cancer is the best thing that ever happened to them.* At first I thought they were kidding, and yet I continued to hear it.

Again, C.P., the woman previously mentioned who had a life-changing experience with God (which included her forgiving a perpetrator of a past pain), wrote, "I can truly, with deep conviction, say, Praise my God, the cancer came back!"

Is she just saying that, or does she really believe it? From my knowledge of her, based on her body language and change in her overall demeanor, I have to say she really believes it.

The idea of thanking God for cancer is a hard sell. And I do not want to diminish anyone's pain and sadness or appear to suggest that anything about cancer treatment, cancer care, and the role faith can play in the healing process is easy to understand or experience. As author Jim Rohn once wrote, "Don't just read the easy stuff. You may be entertained by it, but you will never grow from it."[1] I would ask that you consider the idea that cancer can be a good friend, even though I know it's not easy to do.

With every orientation class I teach at our hospital, I always tell the group of new patients about my goal: to make their cancer experience one of the best things that has ever happened to them. One such day, I found myself sitting across the table from a young breast cancer patient and her husband. She was exhausted after a long day in the clinic undergoing examinations and consultations. After I shared my goal, her husband smiled and nodded. She, on the other hand, said, "I don't think that is possible."

The next day I met her sitting alone in the lobby and struck up a conversation with her. I invited her to my office to see if she had any questions about our conversation the previous day. Before long, she shared that she was very angry about a lot of things. A half-hour later, after sharing much clinical data in conjunction with my pastoral counseling, I said again that I hoped she would see her cancer as one of the best things that had ever happened to her. Specifically, I hoped she would experience the seismic, paradigm-shifting changes that would allow her to view her life and its struggles more positively.

Anger, I said, grows out of feeling powerless. It is the feeling we have when we are not in control of our life and the circumstances we find ourselves living. Some people, I told her, choose to be OK with being powerless. They find themselves relieved at not always having to be in control. It is OK to allow God to be in control of our future (as if we could alter God's plan for our life anyway). For the first time, her eyes widened. It was as though light was beginning to pierce her spiritual defenses. I could almost hear her thinking, *Maybe it's time for me to begin to trust God with my life.*

On the one hand, it would seem hurtful, if not downright cruel, to tell someone who is bravely battling a disease such as cancer that it can be viewed as one of the best things that ever happened to them. And, at any given moment, I might agree. However, here's the problem: Many people I see on a regular basis would say that this is unequivocally true! Cancer, for them, is one of the best things, if not *the* best thing, that has ever happened to them. Further, I believe I can help them come to that realization. To deny anyone that opportunity, especially when he or she is facing a life-threatening disease, seems crueler than suggesting it as a possibility.

With my patients, I will choose the narrow road that leads to life, even though it means that some of my patients will be suspicious of my advice. I work hard to make their cancer experience a wonderful, life-changing, spiritually renewing, emotionally rejuvenating, lifestyle-recalibrating, physically rewarding experience—*if* they want to be healed (John 5:6)—in mind and soul as much as in body.

As I mentioned, when I share this goal with my patients, I am often met with a blank stare, a kind of "deer caught in the headlights" look. However, many nod in agreement—they seem to understand exactly what I mean without my having to say another word. One such gentleman was a sixty-something-year-old man, C.M., who said, "Cancer brings you back to terra firma. I've learned to value each day, instead of taking it for granted. I've also become much closer to my wife."

Another person, J.P., said although she has always been a compassionate person, having cancer has made her reach out to more people. Now that she can personally identify with their pain and worry, she has redoubled her efforts to extend mercy and love. It has given her, she said, "a renewed purpose for living."

Often those who agree with me believe their lifestyle or life decisions contributed to their getting cancer. Therefore, when I suggest that having cancer might be an opportunity for them to regroove their life, they are eager to hear more. Further, they are often motivated and willing students.

One patient was a woman who has been battling breast cancer and its effects for a long time. When I shared my goal (of having this be the most enriching time of her life) she began to cry. I had to scramble down the hall for some tissues.

Then I explained what I meant by my statement. I spoke of the importance of regaining a balance with God. I spoke of learning to trust in God's love, even in the midst of pain and concern. I spoke of the power of prayer and of the miracles I have witnessed.

The reason I shared my experience of the miraculous is because, rightly or wrongly, many people with cancer believe it will take a miracle to save them. I want them to know that if it is a miracle they think they need, a miracle is possible.

Here are a few examples of miracles I've witnessed, and I share them with the hope that you too will find encouragement.

STORIES OF MIRACLES

A ninety-five-year-old woman developed pneumonia, which everyone knows is particularly serious in an elderly person. She had been absent from church for a week or so, and I learned from her friends at her retirement community of her illness. One night I went to her apartment to pray with her. I sat her on her sofa and, after visiting with her for a few minutes, anointed her head with oil and laid my hands right above her lungs. I prayed for God to heal her, if it was his will to do so. Four days later she was back in church! She told me that right after our prayer she began to feel better. She would tell you that God healed her lungs through that prayer.

Similarly, B.G., one of our cancer patients, also had pneumonia, which delayed him from completing his chemotherapy. I placed my hands on his chest and asked God to heal his pneumonia. The next day I was greeted by this same man, who had experienced a dramatic reversal and was scheduled to get his chemo later that day.

Allen S., a dear friend, had a sizable tumor in his stomach that required having two-thirds of his stomach removed. Our church leaders prayed for him. The next day, during surgery, the doctors could not locate the tumor.

Another healing story I like to tell is about my friend Maxine, who has contracted mycobacterium avium, a chronic lung disease. This disease has no cure, and one of its symptoms is that the lungs get darker and darker over time. In the presence of her husband, Bob, I prayed for her. Several days later she visited her doctor, who took X-rays of her lungs. After viewing them he said, "Maxine, what have you been doing?"

"Why?"

"Your upper lobes are almost clear."

"Well, I've been having people pray for me," she said. To which he responded with a catch in his throat, "Would you pray for me? My wife is very ill."

God had caused a dramatic improvement in Maxine's condition. Prayer matters. God continues to amaze us with his grace.

In sharing stories of miracles I've witnessed, I have had very few skeptics. However, in a group setting one day, one such person said I was doing the group a disservice; I was giving them false hope for a miracle. I didn't have to defend myself; the rest of the group did it for me—both directly and indirectly they expressed their opinion. They believe in miracles.

I have many other stories of healing and miracles. I have learned firsthand that beyond the marvelous technology and technicians, machinery and mechanics, there is a God who created it all. And miracles do happen. However, it is our human nature to wonder why some people experience miraculous healing and others do not. We wonder if God's hand of blessing will fall upon the head of our loved one, and if not, why? Ask these questions if you must. Most of us do at one time or another. This is how I addressed the issue recently at a funeral I conducted for one of our cancer patients—a beautiful, smiling wife, loving mother, and dutiful daughter—who didn't survive her disease.

At her funeral, I told those gathered that miracles are a possibility, and I related stories about several I had witnessed. Why, I asked, didn't this wonderful woman receive a miracle? It certainly wasn't because we hadn't asked for one. The only conclusion I could draw was that in the providence of God it was her time to go. Yet, I said, even if God disclosed his reason why he chose to not do a miracle, I was certain that God's reason, at that moment, would be completely unsatisfactory to us. When what we want is our loving wife and mother and daughter back to hold and hug, what reason could there be that would satisfy us? Nevertheless, miracles can and do happen.

If you as a caregiver do not believe in the possibility of amazing things happening in the life of your loved one, perhaps you can use this time to explore what you believe about God and why you believe it. I hope to teach you how to help someone struggling with a chronic or life-threatening disease. Perhaps, along the way, you will be able to say to yourself that cancer is one of the best things that ever happened to you as a caregiver, as well as to your loved one, as together you battle this mean disease.

If cancer can be a positive experience for people who have it, why can't caring for someone with cancer be equally positive? If cancer patients can learn enormously important things about life, why can't their caregivers learn these lessons too? Why can't the time we spend with those who are hurting be a brilliant ray of light against a backdrop of dreary gray?

As one author put it so well,

> There is something I know about you that you may not even know yourself. You have within you more resources of energy than have ever been tapped, more talent than has ever been exploited, more strength than has ever been tested, and more to give than you have ever given.[2]

Together, let's find the energy, the talent, and the strength to give—and then reach out to help a friend in need. Why should we wait to have cancer to learn the marvelous lessons that it may have to teach us?

CHAPTER FIVE

The Roles We Play

---◆---

UNDERLYING THE APPLICATION OF CARE ... IS SINCERITY. WITHOUT SINCERITY
CARING ACTS RING HOLLOW. SINCERE CARE IS REQUIRED TO ACHIEVE A TRUE
SERVICE ATTITUDE WITH PEOPLE. WHEN CARE IS MECHANICAL OR INSINCERE, IT
CAUSES RESISTANCE AND REACTION IN OTHERS, UNDERMINING ADAPTABILITY.
COWORKERS, FAMILY, CLIENTS, AND SUPERIORS CAN TELL THE DIFFERENCE
BETWEEN REQUIRED COURTESY AND SINCERE CARE.

—Doc Childre and Bruce Cryer, *From Chaos to Coherence*

The fact that you are reading this book suggests that you are both caring and sincere. You truly want to help your loved one cope with and overcome his or her disease. To do this, you need to understand that we have many roles to play—peacemaker, life coach, crisis manager, and protector.

PEACEMAKER

The word *medicine* has as its root "med," which is the anglicized version of the Latin root "mid" from which we get the word *middle*. When we find ourselves physically destabilized or out of balance, we are no longer in the middle. We do not experience homeostasis or equilibrium. This is what drives us to the doctor's office. We go seeking to regain balance—to be restabilized—to be at peace. The doctor helps us to find this by offering medicine.

Not to overemphasize the obvious, let's be sure to understand the point: The goal is to return to a balanced, peaceful life. This is what medicine at all levels attempts to help patients do.

Your loved one is experiencing physical disequilibrium, and it is our hope and prayer that your medical team can and will lead your friend back to peace and health. Health-care professionals know, however, that it is very hard, if not impossible, to help people regain physical balance if they are also out of balance spiritually and/or emotionally.

Much has been written about the mind-body connection. Dr. Patrick Quillen, a leading expert in the field of nutrition and its effects on cancer, said, "There is no such thing as a [mind-body] connection, because there never was a disconnection in the first place!"[1] We are seamless human beings. Our minds and bodies are so fully integrated that we are, in essence, one fabric of being.

This is critically important for you to understand and appreciate. It is enormously difficult to make people physically healthy if they are struggling with psychological and/or emotional disorders. In some cases the disease itself may be a physical manifestation of the under-lying emotional or spiritual disorder—a sickness of the soul.

My hospital and I are about to participate in a major study on the relationship between immune-system function and forgiveness. You may wonder why a major cancer treatment hospital would concern itself with issues related to forgiveness, assuming, perhaps, that forgiveness issues ought to be relegated to a person's pastor, rabbi, or priest. Our experience, however, has taught us that people who develop cancer are often dealing with major, untreated psychological and/or emotional wounds. We understand how important it is to help people deal with the emotional traumas they have experienced, because these traumas, such as a divorce, the death of a loved one, or moving cross-country, may be a significant factor in why their body's immune system failed.

Forgiveness begins with a choice to forgive and ends with the return of feelings of positive emotions toward the offender. If you are angry with yourself, know that until you learn to love yourself again you will not have completed the cycle of forgiveness. Jesus, according to the parable of the unmerciful servant (Matt. 18:21–35), made a forgiving heart a prerequisite for entrance into the kingdom of God. Forgive yourself. Forgive others. It should be no surprise that forgiveness, according to Dan Baker, author of the book *What Happy People Know*, is listed as the number one attribute of happy people![2]

Balance. Harmony. Equilibrium. Peace of mind and body and spirit. These are our goals as professional caregivers, and we trust that you will make this a primary goal of your caregiving as well.

LIFE COACH

You and I are not medical coaches. Obviously, we want to help our loved ones make good decisions relative to their health. As a firm believer in second opinions, I don't recommend you always accept every medical conclusion as the last word on the subject. However, I do recommend that you leave medical conclusions to the professionals who have devoted their lives to dealing with cancer and other life-threatening diseases. This creates a dilemma: Whom can you trust? Most of us have barriers limiting our choices such as are defined by insurance coverage and distance to be traveled. My advice to patients who come to my hospital for a second, and sometimes a third, opinion is this: Find a medical team that garners your complete trust. Once you have found your trusted health-care team, trust them with your physical well-being. Don't waste your time worrying about your body—let them take care of you physically. Spend your time doing things that bring you peace and joy.

As caregiver, your primary role is that of a life coach, someone who can help a loved one experience each and every minute as meaningfully, purposefully, and joyfully as possible. As a life coach, you are commissioned to help your loved one fully live, not only during the hospital stay or duration of treatment, but also afterward. A life coach is concerned about the cancer patient's lifestyle in and out of the hospital—from today forward.

Why is it important to show care after treatment ends? Consider this: What benefit have we offered if, after we help our loved ones overcome a battle with cancer, we simply allow them to return to a lifestyle that may have contributed to their disease? Cancer specialists frequently see people return with a recurrence of their cancer, even after the magical five-year period. Why? Perhaps, in part, it is because people sometimes return to toxic lifestyles and environments that contributed to their developing cancer. This is an unfortunate, though common, failure in cancer care and prevention.

For example, I met with one woman in her midthirties who has breast cancer. Her body language and physical demeanor suggested she was peaceful and calm. She shared that things were not going well at home. Her husband seemed to be indifferent about her having cancer.

She said, "He seems to be more interested in when I'm coming home from my chemotherapy than how I'm doing!"

I invited her to write a letter to her husband, sharing with him her frustrations about his behavior—not a letter to be mailed, but shared with me as I helped her process her feelings. The letter I got several days later was very surprising: four pages of utter *rage!* She said that once she began to write, she became flooded with anger. Even she was surprised at how angry she was. Realizing how toxic her marriage had become, she resolved to spend the next few months convalescing with her relatives instead of going back home.

Did her marriage contribute to her getting cancer? I don't know. Maybe. But I'm pretty sure her decision to take care of herself, first and foremost, was a wise and prudent one.

A longtime friend of mine is a top executive for a large pharmaceutical company whose primary business is developing cancer-fighting drugs. I asked him what percentage of patients got cancer due to their genetic makeup rather than environmental and/or sociological reasons. His response was haunting. He said less than 5 percent of people get cancer solely due to their genetic makeup. The logical implication appears to be that 95 percent of cancer may be avoidable!

Of course, there needs to be a word of caution here. It is obvious that we do not easily control our emotions. The way we respond to circumstances is a by-product of lifelong learning. Our coping mechanisms have been honed over the years, and we respond automatically to certain stimuli. When a car slams on its brakes in front of us, our response is immediate. And yet, with help, we can learn to respond differently to situations; we can develop the skills necessary to react in constructive, helpful ways. When that car cuts you off on the highway, there are other options besides road rage. We can develop a healthy attitude to help us cope with negative circumstances, including cancer.

As a life coach, you ought to be concerned about your loved one's physical, emotional, mental, and spiritual habits—habits that may have contributed to the disease. Being a life coach isn't easy, and there is no guarantee you will be able to effect change, but it may be the most rewarding experience of your life.

In some ways life coaching is similar to parenting—it can be difficult, disappointing, and yet, at the same time, personally gratifying. Without clear goals, however, parents won't know if they are successful. When I taught parenting classes throughout the United States and in South Africa, my primary purpose was to help parents learn the goal of parenting. Without a goal and some understanding of what a parent's real purpose ought to be, parenting can be, and often is, a very unrewarding experience.

The same is true for caregiving. Caregiving can be unrewarding, emotionally exhausting, and fraught with all kinds of worries or concerns, many of which may be unavoidable. Without a philosophical or theoretical framework, including the understanding of the goal of caregiving, you may find your experience as a caregiver to be dreadfully laborious and wearisome. In later chapters, I will give you a framework to help you set goals for your loved one.

CRISIS MANAGER

Crises create opportunities for achieving personal growth, enhancing relationships, protecting the vulnerable, guiding the lost and confused, and ensuring your loved one gets needed and deserved care. As Allan K. Chalmers reminds us, "Crises refine life. In them you discover what you are."[3] The kinds of crises caregivers usually face have to do with changes in the loved one's physical well-being. Truth be known, life gets very basic for cancer patients. For example, a daily conversation with medical staff will focus on bowel movements or the lack thereof. People vomit. They lose their hair. Skin sometimes yellows. Weight is lost, often dramatically. Blood counts drop. Pain medications are not always distributed when needed most. Food service is not always on time. There is almost always *something* that is not going right. And there you are right in the middle of it all, facing one crisis after the other. Here's my heartfelt advice: Expect these crises. Learn to be a positive, helpful, nonanxious presence in the midst of them. Do not continually react, or overreact, to them, for if you do, you may well become the next patient.

I am not naive, though admittedly it may seem so. The question caregivers face daily is this: How will I respond to the crises I am going to face today? The lesson I am trying to underscore is this: Your response, if overwhelmingly anxious and negative, may, in the end, be counterproductive. Be, as best you can, a calm presence in the midst of a sea of anxiety.

The crisis created by learning about and having to deal with your friend's infirmity has, I believe, a wonderful advantage to it. You have a marvelous opportunity to enhance your own personal happiness and love for living, to engage or reengage with God at a time when you need him the most, and to learn fundamental truths that are frequently overlooked because of shock and self-pity. Many people never learn to truly live. The fortunate ones are those who have the opportunity to slow down and then take advantage of that slower pace to analyze what is truly important. These people have the chance to reinvent themselves as lovelier, happier, and more self-fulfilled people.

I have encountered a wide range of human needs in my role as pastor. I remember one woman who had experienced many ups and downs in life. Sadly, she continues to repeat the same negative behavioral patterns and has never taken the time to evaluate her approach to life.

It's interesting to note that the word *idiot* comes from the Greek word *idios*, meaning "private." An idiot was someone who was so private that he was unwilling to open himself to learning from other people. Our self-perceptions are limited, and we can learn a lot about ourselves from others. It's also valuable to enlist help from other caregivers who have gone before you and who have found caregiving a wonderful, life-giving vocation. Learn from them, and then share what you learn with your loved one.

All of these opportunities for personal growth are there if you are willing to view cancer or other chronic diseases, not as plagues to be avoided, but as a means to understand how best to care for ourselves and those we love.

PROTECTOR

Isn't it amazing the way people often treat dogs and cats better than human beings? Have you ever wondered why? It's because animals are often more helpless, vulnerable, and defenseless than people. Mistreatment takes place when a protector stops protecting. Protecting all life is important. As Abraham Lincoln once said, "I care not much for a man's religion whose dog and cat are not the better for it." Life in any form is our perpetual responsibility.

The Bible reminds us of our dependence on God's protection. The psalmist wrote, "I am in pain and distress; may your salvation, O God, protect me" (Ps. 69:29).

One of the roles we all play as caregivers is that of protector, particularly from Satan, whose very nature is to destroy life by preying on those who are weak and vulnerable. Here are some things you can protect your loved one from.

BAD MEDICAL CARE

In my view, any doctor who tells you that you have X number of days/weeks/months to live violates the Hippocratic oath to "do no harm." Harvard Medical School reinforces the philosophy that "what you believe is what you become." If a patient believes the doctor who tells the patient he or she has, for example, six weeks to live, it follows that that person's body is going to begin to shut down, making long-term survivability unlikely. Call it self-fulfilling prophecy if you like, but the fact remains that when a person is confronted with a hopeless situation, survival is highly unlikely.

If your doctor gives up on you or your loved one, get another doctor. I have seen people at the brink of death come back strong, especially when they are around people who are hopeful and optimistic. Remember, only "God is in charge of deciding human destiny" (James 4:11 MSG).

BAD SPIRITUAL CARE

Let me define the often-misunderstood term *spirituality*. The word *religion* comes from the conjoining of two Latin words, *re-ligio*, which literally means "re-ligament." The word denotes reconnection and restoration. Theologically we understand that humans are separated from a holy God by sinfulness. Through our "religion" we believe the relationship is "reestablished." Most of the world's religions teach this as a central doctrine.

A person's spirituality is composed of those activities that enable him or her to maintain the vitality of the relationship. Examples include prayer, Scripture reading and study, worship, and participating in rituals such as the Eucharist or Passover meal. Christians also maintain a vital relationship through loving and forgiving their neighbors and enemies. A person's spirituality is not always limited to expressions of his or her own formal religion but is often injected from the culture. For example, regardless of their particular belief system, Americans typically consider "The Battle Hymn of the Republic" or "America the Beautiful" part of their religious and spiritual heritage.

"Bad spiritual care" in a clinical setting is care that ignores or disrespects the patient's relationship with God. It is care that doesn't honor beliefs or provide resources to enable the patient to maintain contact with God.

Let me give you an illustration. One of my patients was convinced God was punishing her by giving her cancer. When asked why she thought this, she told me she was Roman Catholic and divorced and remarried outside the church. When she got cancer, she believed God was getting even for her disregard of the church's teachings.

I could have tried to convince her otherwise by sharing my Protestant views, but my role as a chaplain wasn't to convert her to my way of thinking. Rather I needed to work with her within her own belief system. I called a local priest, shared the situation, and sought his advice. He asked me to tell her God does not give people cancer as a punishment for sin, which I happily did. That little drop of grace changed the woman's demeanor immediately; she also changed physically and spiritually.

In my view, bad spiritual care is care that allows the patient to become sad, despondent, and hopeless without attempting to encourage, uplift, and bring the ministry of joyful living into his or her life. Some patients are by nature unhappy people. Too, some people have been beaten down by years and years of fighting cancer. Nevertheless, my role and yours is to continue to be a source of hope and optimism, an expression of love they can cling to, even when they themselves are unable to muster a smile or focus their attention on positive thoughts.

Bad Treatment Strategy

Many chaplains are trained to *meet the patient where they are*— to enter the patient's world of sadness, anger, or grief in order to acknowledge and validate the patient's feelings. This may be fine if your patient isn't facing a life-threatening disease. But I believe the challenge of chaplaincy, at least for those coping with cancer, has less to do with my meeting patients in their world than them meeting *me* in mine. I don't want to enter a world of sadness. Rather I want to help people enter a world of joy and happiness. I want patients to be as joyful and optimistic as possible, because it is in their best interest to be so. Being joyful is a biblical mandate.

John Templeton put it well when he said, "Happiness comes from spiritual wealth, not material wealth.... Happiness comes from giving, not getting. If we try hard to bring happiness to others, we cannot stop it from coming to us also. To get joy, we must give it, and to keep joy, we must scatter it."[4] And a Chinese proverb expresses it so wonderfully: "If I keep a green bough in my heart, then the singing bird will come."

The challenge for caregivers, particularly those helping someone facing life-threatening disease, is to keep the green bough of joy, care, and appreciation in our hearts, trusting that as we do, our loved ones will find a good place to rest—a healing place.

NEGATIVITY

Protect your loved one from slipping into self-pity and despair by helping him or her regain their focus—help the person. Mark Twain cleverly wrote, "The best way to cheer yourself up is to try to cheer somebody else up."[5]

Depression and sadness not only diminish the efforts of the rest of the health-care team, but also reflect an unhealthy and unhelpful belief system. It is one thing to visit and care for the sick, it is quite another to contribute to their disease through your own negativity. Show me a sad chaplain and I'll show you a chaplain who doesn't understand the essence of the good news or believe in the biblical doctrine of the providence of God. Show me a pastoral-care team whose goal is to "meet people where they are" and I'll show you a pastoral-care team that may not fully appreciate the healing power of hope.

I am not suggesting insensitivity, although I admit that it may sound that way. I understand the importance of creating a pastoral relationship with someone by gaining understanding and exhibiting respect. I also believe, however, those who care for patients with cancer and other life-threatening diseases need to be aware that time is of the essence; what is needed is "spiritual triage," ministry that explodes with hope, optimism, and joy. This kind of caregiving can only be administered by caregivers who are themselves hopeful, optimistic, and joyful. Even in the face of death, if we believe in a sovereign God and his promises, we can find a reason to be joyful.

If you or your loved one is struggling with issues related to religion or spirituality, if you wonder, in light of pain and disease, whether or not God even exists, I invite you to consider this poem titled *Faith* by David Whyte:

> I want to write about faith
> About the way the moon rises
> Over cold snow, night after night
>
> Faithful even as it fades from fullness
> Slowly becoming that last curving and impossible
> Sliver of light before the final darkness
> But I have no faith myself
> I refuse to give it the smallest entry
>
> Let this then, my small poem
> Like a new moon, slender and barely open
> Be the first prayer that opens me to faith.[6]

POOR JUDGMENT

Poor medical care, in my view, is medical care that leaves a patient devoid of hope. Every form of cancer, even at its latest stages, has been survived. Therefore removing a person's hope seems cruel and heartless. It is one thing for a doctor to tell a patient there is nothing more that the hospital can do for them. It is quite another to tell them nothing can be done at all. Poor *judgment*, on the other, takes seriously the reality that reasonable people can differ on treatment options. For example, a medical oncologist who denigrates the benefits of holistic health care, such as the importance of nutrition, spiritual care, naturopathy, and mind/body medicine is simply exercising poor judgment. That is why I suggest that, if possible, patients should seek a second opinion. Why? Although there may be a consensus by the medical community as to how to treat certain forms of cancer, it is also true that there are so many new drugs and treatment therapies that it is worth the effort to compare treatment plans. Cancer treatments are often similar, but often not. For example, sometimes one oncologist will insist on a combination of chemotherapy and radiation, while another will be satisfied with one or the other. Many people seek a second opinion and often a third, so don't think it is at all unusual.

PASSIVITY

Many cancer patients are passive about their disease. Often it is the caregiver who initiates contact with our hospital. Now is the time to *fight* disease with *gentle confidence* in God and the health-care team assembled to treat the patient. You as the caregiver may need to be the one who actively pursues options.

UNFAIR INSURANCE PRACTICES

It's common practice for insurance companies to automatically deny coverage, particularly when it comes to paying larger claims. They know a certain percentage of patients will not resubmit a claim, which of course allows them to remain profitable as well as keep insurance premiums lower. However, consider this real-life situation: A woman was denied coverage for a stem-cell procedure costing $30,000. After months of submitting requests for coverage, her husband was finally granted a face-to-face meeting with the insurance company's case manager. The case manager felt sorry for the man and told him the truth. She said his policy did not cover all of the $30,000 dollars that was being requested. It only covered $25,000, so the claim was rejected in whole. She told the man that if he could come up with the additional $5,000, she would fund the $25,000.

He had been wading for months through a sea of red tape while his wife suffered needlessly. The insurance company didn't offer to pay the $25,000 until the husband finally connected with a compassionate human being.

I spoke with a friend of mine who is an executive with one of the world's largest insurance companies. He told me, off the record, that this is common practice in the insurance field. Frightening! Protect your loved one from insensitive insurance practices. Resubmit. Resubmit again. And try to see your case manager if you are not satisfied with your results.

Among the various roles that caregivers play, these are the most important:

- Peacemaker
- Life Coach
- Crisis Manager
- Protector

As every pastor knows: If you can't name the sin, you can't tame the sin. The same is true for caregiving: If you can't name the roles, you can't play them. As the 1974 Nobel Laureate Linus Pauling, PhD, taught us,

> The optimum treatment of the cancer patient requires a concerted multidisciplinary approach employing the full resources of surgery, radiotherapy, chemotherapy, immunotherapy and supportive care. The last named has received the least attention, although it may well possess great potential for therapeutic advance.[7]

Remember that as you share your love and care with a patient, you are not only contributing to the person's well-being, you are playing an important and integral role on the health-care team. As a candle of hope, you may be the most influential member of the team.

CHAPTER SIX

Be a Real Friend

—————— ❖ ——————

A REAL FRIEND IS ONE WHO WALKS IN
WHEN THE REST OF THE WORLD WALKS OUT.

—Walter Winchell

IF ONE FALLS DOWN,

HIS FRIEND CAN HELP HIM UP.

BUT PITY THE MAN WHO FALLS

AND HAS NO ONE TO HELP HIM UP!

—Ecclesiastes 4:10

It really is true that you find out who your friends are when you need them the most. True friends are there for you, often without asking. When you are scheduled for surgery, true friends are there to provide care, support, and prayer. When you find out you have cancer, true friends are not frightened by the diagnosis. They may not know what to do or say, but they refuse to allow their inadequacies to keep them away. As the Scriptures remind us, "Friends love through all kinds of weather" (Prov. 17:17 MSG).

I admire the special people—family members, close friends, or old friends from high school—who put their lives on hold to help someone they love. Emotional and spiritual ties bind people together in supernatural ways.

It is also important to note that there are good friends who, for whatever reason, cannot be there for a loved one during times of great need. These friends will still make their caring concern known in other ways, by sending cards and letters or making unexpected phone calls.

But many people don't have as much control over time as they would like to think they do. Responsibilities to others cannot always be put aside. Just because key friends are unable to be there for a patient doesn't mean that they don't care deeply.

Real friends walk in—whether it's close at hand or from a distance—and you've walked in. Good for you. And may God bless your efforts.

REAL FRIENDS CARRY BURDENS

Caring for others is a noble virtue. Its nobility is one of the reasons why people tend to hold medical doctors in such high regard. However noble it may be, you and I, as people of faith, understand that caring for others is an obligation placed on us as part of our spiritual heritage. Consider this imperative: "If anyone does not provide for his relatives, and especially for his immediate family, he has denied the faith and is worse than an unbeliever" (1 Tim. 5:8).

Remember the parable of the good Samaritan? It's a familiar story. Our society even has "Good Samaritan" laws to protect those who risk helping someone in need. Early in the Old Testament, God was angered by Cain's treatment of Abel (Gen. 4:9–16). Cain had not learned a basic truth: We are our "brother's keeper."

The Scriptures are packed with encouragement to care for others during times of need. Paul wrote in Galatians 6:2, "Carry each other's burdens, and in this way you will fulfill the law of Christ."

Old Testament prophets, such as Isaiah, teach us that we have an obligation to help others: "Is not this the kind of fasting I have chosen: to loose the chains of injustice and untie the cords of the yoke, to set the oppressed free and break every yoke?" (Isa. 58:6).

Surely most of us already understand the moral imperative we have to help others, particularly those who are vulnerable, such as widows or orphans (James 1:27), or those who have experienced illness or other tragic circumstances. Knowing we have a responsibility to help isn't the problem for us—knowing what to do and how to do it is the difficulty.

Most of us feel inadequate, and thus we don't always want to accept our responsibility. So we turn the caregiving over to another family member or friend.

I once met a woman who was receiving chemotherapy for breast cancer. She had become the primary caregiver for her aging and very needy mother. Because she lived relatively close to her, she was willing to spend a lot of time providing for her. Caring for an aging parent is stressful, and because stress is a primary cause for immune system malfunction, taking care of her mother may have contributed to the woman's developing breast cancer.

Her situation was even more tragic because she had several brothers and sisters who lived closer to her mother than she did, and yet *she* became the primary caregiver, while her siblings did little for their mother.

Caregiving can be difficult. And it can be as unrewarding as it is difficult. We sometimes feel taken for granted and unappreciated. There's not a parent, teacher, therapist, preacher, doctor, or nurse in the world who would disagree with that statement. Emotional, psychological, and spiritual pitfalls go hand in hand with helping others.

The question is, why is it so difficult? Why so unrewarding? Is there anything that can be done to make it more life-giving and enjoyable? The answer to the last question is an unequivocal *yes!* I will explain later how to make it so. But even when caregiving is more enjoyable, it still isn't easy, just easier.

REAL FRIENDS BRING JOY

The caregiving philosophy I offer in this book I refer to as "joy-based" caregiving because I believe life at its best is lived joyfully.

I don't believe joy and happiness are limited to exciting and pleasurable moments. Joy can be experienced even during the most oppressive circumstances.

Victor Frankl, a Holocaust survivor, wrote about his horrific experiences in a Nazi concentration camp in his book *Man's Search for Meaning.* "Everything can be taken from a man but one thing: the last of the human freedoms—to choose one's attitude in any given set of circumstances, to choose one's own way."[1] He developed a method of psychology he named "logotherapy," in which he states his belief that suffering is not an obstacle to happiness but often the necessary means to it, less a pathology than a path. Further, what logotherapy amounts to is the advice "Get to work." Other psychologies begin by asking, "What do I want from life? Why am I unhappy?" Logotherapy asks, "What does life at this moment demand of me?"

Frankl's theory suggests that joy and happiness are desirable emotional states regardless of situation or circumstances. This coincides with what the Scriptures teach us: "Be joyful always; pray continually; give thanks in all circumstances, for this is God's will for you in Christ Jesus" (1 Thess. 5:16–18).

Happiness and joy are not easy to obtain, and so we spend a great deal of energy, money, and other resources in pursuit of them. Yet happiness and joy continue to elude us even though we know they are God's will for us.

It is fundamentally impossible to worry while at the same time trusting in God. Complete trust in God dissipates worry; they are mutually exclusive.

The same holds true for happiness and anxiety. While we are experiencing happiness it is impossible to be overwhelmed with negative feelings. This is especially important news for people battling immune-system diseases such as cancer and HIV/AIDS. To the extent I am able to relieve patients from anxiety, worry, and stress, I am enabling their immune system to function at a higher level. But more importantly, I am helping people live life as God intended it to be lived.

Being joyful and happy, therefore, ought to be the highest priority for cancer patients. And if it is their highest priority, it ought also to be their caregiver's priority. As the Scriptures remind us, "A happy heart makes the face cheerful, but heartache crushes the spirit" (Prov. 15:13), and as Lincoln quipped, "Most people are about as happy as they make up their minds to be."

Caregivers need to make up their minds to be happy so cheerfulness can be multiplied in the lives of those they love and care for. And here's another noteworthy thought: "According to happiness research, choosing [i.e., the ability to make choices] feels better than almost anything."[2]

If a Holocaust survivor such as Victor Frankl can choose to find meaning, purpose, and happiness in the midst of the most horrific of all human experiences, you and I can help those we love to do the same. However, remember, you can't motivate the unmotivated. There are some people for whom the glass is always half empty and for whom the roses never seem to be fragrant. Nevertheless, we can try.

REAL FRIENDS BRING HOPE

Both patients and caregivers frequently ask this question: Is there such a thing as false hope? My answer is, "Of course! Any time anyone tells you that you have X number of days, weeks, months, or years to live, they have given you false hope." Why? Because no one knows how long anyone is going to live. There are no guarantees. Some people with stage 4 cancer may very well outlive me. Conversely, some well-meaning oncologist may tell the stage 4 cancer patient that he or she has six weeks to live, eventually to discover the patient didn't make it through the week or lived thirty more years. No one knows how long anyone is going to live, except God.

Please do not think I'm trivializing the seriousness of your loved one's disease. I know how precious this life is and how quickly it can be taken away. All the more reason to enjoy every minute of life we are given to live.

I fervently want every cancer patient and critically ill person I am privileged to care for to find their experience filled with hope and joy, an experience they will cherish and remember after their hospital departure. I hope to help them discover a new way of living—a lifestyle of abundant living for the remainder of their days. When visitors happen upon an outpatient cancer clinic that I oversee, I want them to be amazed at the joy and cheerfulness on the faces of the patients, staff, and caregivers.

I'm not asking you to make a room full of cancer patients happy; I'm asking you to help make just one of them happy: your loved one, for I want you to be a dreamer of dreams and a pursuer of hope and happiness, even during difficult times. It is my dream and my prayer for you that you will not let cancer steal the joy from your heart.

The goal of caregiving is to create a physical and emotional environment where, in spite of the possibility of death, the order of the day is joy, not sadness. Hope, not despair. Life and living, not fear of death and dying.

REAL FRIENDS RESPECT A PATIENT'S RIGHT TO ENJOY LIFE

Cancer patients have the right to be happy as they face an uncertain future. They have the right to live out their life, however long it is, with joy, laughter, accomplishment, and purpose. The job of a caregiver is to ensure our loved ones are aware of the choices they have to experience joy or sadness—and then, assuming they prefer joy over sadness, to help them learn to be and stay joyful. How? By our joyful example!

As a caregiver, especially to cancer patients, resist the temptation to focus on how long your loved one might live. Remember that *no one* knows the answer to "How long?" but God. What we do know about life, for all of us, is that it is fleeting.

Show me, O LORD, my life's end
and the number of my days;
let me know how fleeting is my life.

You have made my days a mere handbreadth;
the span of my years is as nothing before you.
Each man's life is but a breath. (Ps. 39:4–5)

We know that life is like a mist. "Why, you do not even know what will happen tomorrow. What is your life? You are a mist that appears for a little while and then vanishes" (James 4:14).

As Jesus taught, "Who of you by worrying can add a single hour to his life?" (Matt. 6:27). We have little control over the quantity of our days; therefore, we ought to focus on those things that bring quality to our life. Life is too fleeting to waste it.

I know you may be thinking that caregiving is easier said than done. And yet, once people are reconciled to the fact that they are mortal and that death cannot be avoided, a supernatural sense of peace and joy often enters their lives. Some of the happiest people I know are people who have cancer. They are not happy *because* they have cancer, they are happy in spite of it. They, better than most of us, have a very high "get it" factor. They get that life is precious. They get that life is temporary. They get the idea that life is not to be wasted. Cancer has forced them into a reality that ultimately leads them to discover what life is about and how they could and should have been living all along. As their caregiver, we are called to help them learn these lessons. But first we need to learn them ourselves.

A life well lived is not filled with regret. That's true for both those dealing with terminal disease and their caregivers. Even if your loved one has little time to live, you will likely regret it if you have not done everything you can to enhance his or her quality of life while you have the opportunity. Remember that this person's life at this (and every) point is in God's hands.

REAL FRIENDS OFFER EMPATHY AND SYMPATHY

If you are a parent, teacher, doctor, nurse, pastor, priest, or a friend who has assumed, to one degree or another, the responsibility of caring for another human being, you know how burdensome and often unrewarding helping others can be. It can be exhausting and life draining. Like me, most of my colleagues go to bed early, fatigued by their service to their patients. Feeling overwhelmed and exhausted is one of the potential side effects of caregiving. I cannot rid myself of these feelings, nor do I want to. Why? Because compassionate, patient-centered caregiving requires both empathy and sympathy, which can be exhausting. It is impossible to be fully present with a suffering patient and not be affected by it.

Although various attempts have been made to define the word *empathy* (the Greek word suggests "entering into pain"), it is qualitatively different than sympathy (shared pain). One helpful source defines empathy as an "intellectual and emotional awareness and understanding of another person's thoughts, feelings, and behavior, even those that are distressing and disturbing. Empathy emphasizes understanding; sympathy emphasizes sharing of another person's feelings and experiences."[3]

Patients want their caregivers to feel empathy—to understand who they are and what they are going through, but they also want them to be sympathetic—to share, to one degree or another, their hurt and pain. In fact, Christians would argue that God, in taking on flesh in Jesus Christ, chose to go beyond merely empathizing with a broken world. He sympathized with it by entering into the human experience, where he chose not to maintain emotional distance from people. Jesus, for example, touched the sick. He wept. He suffered. He not only understood people's disease and pain, but also entered into it.

REAL FRIENDS GET IN THE DITCH

A useful metaphor I was taught in seminary is that of trying to help a person who is "in a ditch." The best way to help someone out of the ditch is not to get into the ditch with them (sympathy) but rather to lend a helpful hand from outside of the ditch (empathy). The reason is obvious: It is difficult to help someone out of the ditch if we caregivers are in the ditch ourselves.

The practical application of this metaphor, however, creates distance.

Caregivers begin to feel the pain, fear, anxiety, hopelessness, powerlessness, and anger of our friends through emotional osmosis. This is one of the risks patient-centered care exposes us to. We do not idly and dispassionately distance ourselves from these uncomfortable feelings, but rather we allow ourselves to hazard the dangerous and often foreign emotional landscape that our friends have learned to call home.

Patient-centered care requires both understanding our patient's needs and personally identifying with them. Many medical professionals see only a person with a disease; after all, this is what the study of medicine requires and what years of experience teach. But sympathy? Holding a hand, listening to someone's story, slowing down to be mentally present with a patient? Empathy does not invariably lead to sympathy, and understanding does not always lead to friendship and love. As Edmund Burke once wrote, "Next to love, sympathy is the divinest passion of the human heart."[4]

I wonder why Burke considered sympathy the "divinest passion." Perhaps it's because it is so rare! Regardless of its rarity, or reasons for it, I have a private conversation with most every patient at the hospital usually lasting thirty minutes or so. I earnestly and sincerely convey to them that I understand their concerns and fears. I truly "get it." But I also tell them that I refuse to pity them. Rather, I tell them, it is my joyful obligation to lift their spirits, to find ways to bring smiles to their faces, joy to their hearts, and words of thanksgiving to their lips. I get in the ditch with them for thirty minutes and then make my way out in order to lead them out of despair into a happier and more hopeful future.

REAL FRIENDS HAVE A GOOD CRY

If you are contemplating the possibility of losing someone you love, you know your heart may be broken in the process. Bad news forces us to deal with a new reality and accept that life has changed and will never be the same regardless of what the future holds.

I know what it feels like to walk with a friend who is hurting, fearful, lonely, and sad. I know the constellation of emotions and feelings and thoughts that, at times, overwhelm us with sorrow. I know what it is like to wonder if my friend will ever again be whole and happy and experience the fullness of human joy and love. I know what it is like to worry about never again seeing someone I love very much—losing them forever and pondering life without their touch, their gentleness, and their sense of humor. After all, in a cancer hospital, we often feel like we are part of the patient's family.

The possibility of tears is the price we pay for loving another human being. Tears validate our care and concern and visibly reflect the myriad of intangible emotions that run, like deep rivers, through us all. Tears are not evidence of weakness, but the overflow of a loving heart. Further, I've learned that in the presence of extraordinary pain and/or sheer exhaustion, it is almost impossible to be positive. As hopeful as we might be for long-term cure, sometimes tears, involuntary and uncontrollable, come flowing.

Feelings such as these are part of the risk we take in loving other human beings. We risk being hurt by their occasional thoughtlessness. We risk feeling lonely when they are not around, and we risk great suffering at the thought of losing them forever. However, we gain from being uplifted by their small successes or casual compliments.

Even the possibility of losing our friend to death or distance causes us to begin a mourning process. So if you are feeling overwhelmed by the possibility of losing your friend or loved one, you are not alone. All of us—the doctors, nurses, chaplains, and everyone else who is a part of your loved one's caregiving team—mourn and grieve with you as you consider the possibility of your loss.

We caregivers should not divorce themselves from our feelings, yet those feelings can also mislead us—they can cause us to give up hope for a longer, stronger relationship and life. Go ahead and grieve and mourn your friend's situation. Cry. Release the emotions that attend the possibility of permanent loss, but remember that life brings hope. It is against the backdrop of the sadness we face at the possibility of losing a loved one that I want to introduce you to hope and joy.

Real Friends Are Often Emotional Sponges

Imagine a sponge lying on your kitchen sink, dry as a bone. Suddenly you become aware of a puddle on the counter. Without thinking, you pick up the sponge and blot up the puddle. The wetness has disappeared, right? Not really. The moisture now resides in the sponge, not on the counter. The wetness has only been relocated from the counter onto the sponge.

This, quite often, is what takes place with people who are kind and compassionate. They are emotional sponges predisposed to soak up other people's problems, and, if they are not careful, also their pain.

Perhaps one of the reasons many physicians are leaving medical practice, besides issues related to malpractice insurance, is that modern methods of patient care require them to be more personally involved with their patients—to be more sympathetic and spend more time with the patient at bedside or during office visits. Doctors experience compassion fatigue like everyone else.

According to one source for medical professionals, burnout is a cumulative process leading to emotional exhaustion and withdrawal. It warns that when you feel a distinct loss of energy and motivation and a sense of paralysis about what to do about it, you may be spiraling into burnout.[5]

If a doctor can experience burnout, so can you. It's hard to imagine that as much as you love the one you're caring for, you might find yourself becoming angry, blowing up, or blaming others for your situation. Some people get depressed. Some withdraw. Others cope with their burnout through drug abuse or other unhelpful coping mechanisms.

Please don't let this discourage you from caregiving. Rather determine to chart a life-giving and emotionally beneficial course. Pace yourself. Take care of your own needs, even if it means leaving your loved one alone for a while. Make sure you are eating well, getting exercise, drinking plenty of water, and getting plenty of rest. You need to take care of yourself, and as you do, you serve as a helpful role model to your friend. You will not do much good for your friend if you break down in the process of taking care of him or her.

The Internet is a wonderful resource for caregiving tips. Consider these self-care tips from Caring Connection's Caringinfo.org:

- **Take a break from caregiving.** Even if it is only fifteen or twenty minutes a day, make sure you do something just for you.
- **Exercise.** Most experts recommend at least thirty minutes, three times a week. This is a great way to take a break, decrease stress, and enhance your energy.
- **Eat healthy.** To help give you more energy, avoid foods that are high in saturated fats, sugar, salts, chemical preservatives and additives, and calories. Your health and nutrition is just as important as the person's you are caring for, so take the time to eat three nutritious meals a day. If you have having difficulty do that, ask for help and get others to fix meals for you.
- **Subscribe to caregiving newsletters or Listservs for advice and support.**
- **Attend a support group for caregivers.** Check with your doctor, hospice, or another community resource for help. See also Family Caregiver 101 (www.familycaregiving101.org) for more about caregiver support groups.
- **Seek professional help.** Many caregivers have times when they are lonely, anxious, guilty, angry, scared, frustrated, confused, lost, and tired. If you feel like these feelings are overwhelming you, call your doctor, hospice, or another community resource (see below) for help.

Other Web sites that I have found personally very helpful are

- Ourjourneyofhope.com
- Christiancancercare.com
- Familydoctor.org
- Bymyside.com
- Cancercaregiving.com
- Caregiver.com

For those of you who would like the benefit of a personal "cancer coach," I would recommend considering the following: acancercoach.com. Dennis Gibson is a patient as well as a cancer coach, and with his theological training as a professor at Wheaton College, you might find his advice to be helpful at many levels.

More than making you aware of the emotional risks and psychological implications of caregiving, I want you to understand that patient-centered caregiving is a door that swings both ways. You can and will soak up some of the patient's pain, worries, and concerns. However, your friend can soak up your feelings as well. Your joy can bring him or her joy. Your positive attitude can and will bring hope and strength to fight the disease. If, by osmosis, your friend's pain can pour into your heart and soul, in turn your personal happiness can flow into his or hers. Your loved one can blot up your happiness the same way you blot up his or her pain.

It is easy to be sad and melancholy around sick people. Visit any hospital or cancer treatment center and you're likely to see sad, depressed patients and staff. You'll see treatment rooms that are dark and lifeless, places where the air is noxious and the sights and sounds gloomy.

What does your demeanor convey to your friend? Are you stretching yourself to feel your friend's pain? Are you stretching yourself in your effort to be happy, knowing your attitude can and will have a positive effect on your friend or loved one? Is your joy pouring into his or her heart and making glad your friend's life at a time he or she most needs to feel happy?

Taking care of yourself means resisting the temptation to succumb to the doubt, disappointment, and despair your friend may be feeling. It is good to connect at that level but not good for either of you to stay there.

REAL FRIENDS RELIEVE STRESS

Of the several subjects you will need to become an expert on, stress is probably at the top of the list. Why? Because stress is a leading cause of immune system malfunction. The more you learn about stress, the better you will be able to help your loved one cope with his or her stress, particularly if your friend is struggling with a disease related to poor immune function.

According to Dr. Herbert Benson, MD, of Harvard Medical School, 60 to 90 percent of people see their primary care physicians because of stress-related diseases. Stress is terribly debilitating.

One organization committed to helping people learn how to cope with life's stresses and strains can be found at www.stressless.com. I recommend that you visit the Web site and learn about stress. Consider taking their online "stress test." The organization offers this list of coping levels to consider:

1. **Stressed Out/Burned Out**. Severe difficulties in coping, incapacitating feelings of anxiety, dread, depression, helplessness and/or anger, impaired functioning on the job or in personal life, extreme distress, presence of physical symptoms such as sleep and/or appetite disturbance, lowered immunity, physical tension, or depleted energy.
2. **Strained.** Frequent difficulty in coping, a sense of being overwhelmed or feeling drained, persistent feelings of anxiety, anger, irritability, helplessness, worry, gloom, some impairment in functioning at work or personal life.
3. **Balanced.** Effective and relatively stable functioning at work and/or personal life. Occasional distressing feelings that are appropriate and minimally disturbing or disruptive.

4. Highly Effective. Highly effective and creative problem solving and performance, feeling challenged, energized, motivated, and anticipating successful resolution.[6]

My hope is that you will be able to provide care for your loved one in a highly effective way. You will not be helpful to anyone if you are feeling overwhelmed, strained, or burned out.

During my seminary training, ministerial candidates were taught, as a highest priority, to take care of themselves. Why? Because we were told if we didn't, no one would. Parish ministry can be very stressful and overwhelming. No wonder there is such an emphasis on personal caretaking.

Another aspect of this involves the ability to be a role model of the Christian life. How can I teach my congregation to live a well-balanced life if I am abusing myself through poor personal habits and engaging in at-risk behaviors?

One of the challenges you will have is learning how stress affects your loved one, while at the same time learning to monitor its effects on you. Several studies suggest that "a supportive person during stressful events can minimize stress, whereas a nonsupportive person can exacerbate the stress."[7] If you are not handling your own stress well, the care you give your friend will be less helpful.

The Institute of HeartMath has developed a program called Freeze-Frame: One Minute Self-Management. They believe it is a "fast-acting power tool for transforming stressful thoughts and emotions into clarity, allowing you to take efficient and effective action. With practice, you gain increased power to come to balance and quickly change a negative, draining response into a proactive, creative one."[8]

If this is true, and my personal experience suggests that it is, the implications for both the patient and caregiver are enormous. Consider the five steps involved in the Freeze-Frame method of stress relief:

1. Take a time out so you can temporarily disengage from your thoughts and feelings, especially stressful ones.
2. Shift your focus to the area around your heart—feel your breath coming in through your heart and out through your solar plexus. Practice breathing this way a few times to ease into the technique.
3. Make a sincere effort to activate a positive feeling. This can be a genuine feeling of appreciation or care for someone, some place, or some thing in your life.
4. Ask yourself what would be an efficient, effective attitude or action that would balance and de-stress your system.
5. Quietly sense any change in perception or feeling and sustain it as long as you can. Heart perceptions are often subtle. Then gently suggest effective solutions that would be best for you and all concerned.[9]

According to HeartMath's research, it can take less than one minute for highly motivated people to relax and gain wonderful physiological benefits. This requires special training and a commitment to your personal well-being. But it's not something everyone can do with equal ease. Some people are so disconnected from their feelings that they truly aren't even aware that they are feeling stress—at least they are unaware of its symptoms.

For years I would get a stiff neck and relieve the stiffness by tilting my head back and forth, which often would cause it to "pop." It's hard to imagine that I never really connected the stiffness with stress. Seems even foolish to confess it, yet there you have it. What, me, worry? Apparently I did, and the pain in my neck was the logical physical consequence of the stress in my life.

Eric Hoffer wrote, "No one is truly literate who cannot read his own heart." I'm not the only person who has had to learn how to "read [my] own heart." Many people experience contractions or a tightening in their chest, sweaty hands, or increased heart rate and are either unaware of it or do not realize the detrimental impact of stress on their body. Anyone who has been separated from a loved one for an extended period knows what a broken heart feels like, that unmistakable viselike pain our hearts can experience. Yet, not everyone who feels the pain of heartsickness seeks a remedy.

Most people do not attempt to regularly relieve the pain, much less take one minute several times a day to alleviate its symptoms. We'll take an aspirin in the morning. We'll take a sleeping pill at night without realizing that our sleep might very well be compromised by unresolved stress. We'll take Prozac or other antidepressants, often without paying attention to some of the underlying causes. We often treat the symptoms but just as often neglect to cure the problem.

The challenge for you and me as caregivers is to be aware of the stress in our lives and the lives of those we love and then deal with it. If we are trying to discover ways to shorten the "space between the notes" (as I will cover in chapter 12), what better way is there to do that than by monitoring our body for signs of stress and then practicing the Freeze-Frame method or other helpful stress management techniques? It is extremely important that we be proactive in the self-management of the stressors in our lives.

REAL FRIENDS REDUCE DEPRESSION THROUGH QUALITY PASTIME MANAGEMENT

Although more will be said about this later, I want to introduce the concept of "pastime management" to prepare you to engage more effectively with this critically important topic. Here is the truth: Time is precious, and for each of us it is growing shorter and shorter. Therefore, we ought to be sure we're using our time as best we can. Unfortunately, it's an easy resource to squander.

In some ways, time is the most important resource we have. It's as common as the air we breathe; however, many of us pollute the air by wasting our time. Consider some thoughts by others who have contemplated time.

Now is the only time there is. Make your now *wow*, your minutes *miracles*, and your days *pay*. Your life will have been magnificently lived and invested, and when you die you will have made a difference.

— MARK VICTOR HANSEN

Time is the coin of your life. It is the only coin you have, and only you can determine how it will be spent. Be careful lest you let other people spend it for you.

— CARL SANDBURG

Minutes are worth more than money. Spend them wisely.

— THOMAS P. MURPHY

The bad news is time flies. The good news is you're the pilot.

— MICHAEL ALTHSULER

Lost time is never found again.

— BENJAMIN FRANKLIN

Probably the most common side effect of cancer is depression. The problem isn't that we (or our loved ones) get depressed. Who doesn't from time to time? The problem is most of us don't know how to cope with it.

Often medical professionals assume the primary treatment for depression is pharmacological—prescribing drugs as the antidote for everything. And while antidepressants have their role in health care, the quickest way to recover is by simply building an action plan for the day—hour by hour, day by day—filling our time with meaningful and interesting things to do.

In the next few chapters I'll say more about this, but its importance cannot be overstated: Make every minute count through planning. A mind given the opportunity to drift will always drift toward negativity and despair.

Every morning, create an action plan or to-do list. Writing goals down doesn't mean you will accomplish everything on the list, but it does increase the likelihood that you might accomplish important activities. Without some level of intentionality, hours can slip into days, weeks, months, and years; important tasks are left undone and life becomes a little less satisfying.

For your own well-being, every morning ask yourself these questions:

- What can I do today to lift my friend's spirits?
- What information does my friend need from me today, and how can I best communicate it?
- What can I do to help my friend experience the presence of God today?
- What aspects of my life are out of balance and need attention?
- Am I fatigued? What am I going to do about it?
- What am I going to do with my time today?

If we try to identify the answers to some or all of these questions, good things will happen. A loved one who is facing a life-threatening disease needs your help to ensure that however much time he or she has left is not thoughtlessly wasted, but rather well spent in activities that bring the person—and you—joy.

Among other things, real friends carry burdens, demonstrate care, bring joy and hope, respect a patient's right to enjoy life, offer empathy and sympathy, get in the ditch with their friend, have a good cry and are emotional sponges, relieve stress, and reduce depression through quality pastime management.

But most importantly, real friends walk in when the rest of the world walks out. Aren't you amazing! You've walked in. Congratulations! While you are there, may God use your ministry of joyful caregiving in mighty, mighty ways.

You, dear reader, are a real friend to the person you are caring for. Thank God for you!

CHAPTER SEVEN

When It's Hard to Focus

❖

AS THE DEER PANTS FOR STREAMS OF WATER,

SO MY SOUL PANTS FOR YOU, O GOD.

MY SOUL THIRSTS FOR GOD, FOR THE LIVING GOD.

WHEN CAN I GO AND MEET WITH GOD?

MY TEARS HAVE BEEN MY FOOD

DAY AND NIGHT,

WHILE MEN SAY TO ME ALL DAY LONG,

"WHERE IS YOUR GOD?"

—Psalm 42:1–3

A close reading of Psalm 42 displays its author, David, as being depressed. He's tearful, feeling abandoned by God and friends. His primary spiritual condition is simple: He is depressed because he has lost his focus in life; he's become disconnected from his purpose for living.

Undoubtedly he knew God is always present. He testified to that fact in Psalm 139, when he wrote, "Where can I go from your Spirit? Where can I flee from your presence? If I go up to the heavens, you are there; if I make my bed in the depths, you are there" (vv. 7–8).

The difference between the two psalms is that when he wrote Psalm 42 he was depressed; his mind became confused. In Psalm 139, he is once again thinking clearly.

Here's the point: The most common experience of typical cancer patients is depression, during which time they are miserable. They often feel angry, lonely, and forsaken by God, friends, and family. They are Psalm 42 people.

Antidepressants are commonly distributed to cancer patients, and though I know medication can be helpful, I wonder if there isn't a better way. My years of working with cancer patients have led me to believe that the quickest and best antidote to depression is regaining focus.

The problem is not "chemo-brain."

It is difficult to maintain focus, even during the best of times. Life's many responsibilities are forever causing us to put today on hold while we plan for tomorrow. Computers, phones, radios, and televisions are often distracting, making the ability to focus on one particular task for any length of time a challenge.

Have you ever thought about your ability to concentrate? What effect does hearing or experiencing bad news or tragedy have on your emotions? Can you think clearly? How would you respond to the news that you have been diagnosed with cancer? Or that your child is missing? Or that you've lost your job? After an emotional lightning bolt rips, tears, and claws its way into your heart, are you easily able to focus on anything for any length of time?

We like to think we could maintain our ability to mentally and emotionally cope with life's problems and difficulties. It seems logical that a person who learns he or she has cancer would begin to focus on the disease and nothing else. But experience in working with cancer patients has taught me otherwise. Cancer patients, in general, often find it difficult to concentrate on anything for more than a handful of moments. In fact, the mind-set of many, if not most, cancer patients parallels those who suffer from attention deficit disorder.

Much has been written about the mental side effects of chemotherapy. One such side effect is often labeled "chemo-brain." This condition is often prevalent long before chemotherapy treatments, however. The problem is not chemo-brain, although chemotherapy may exacerbate the problem. The problem is not "pain-brain," although the side effects of pain medication may also complicate the problem. The problem is that cancer patients are often emotionally overwhelmed by all they have to deal with, all the issues that affect their ability to process information. Thoughts become moving targets.

Over the years I've asked cancer patients about their ability to concentrate, and virtually everyone agrees it has been significantly diminished. Heads nod when I ask them if they struggle to maintain their ability to focus. Here's the problem: The ability to concentrate is an essential ingredient for happiness!

Consider this list of things patients have to think about:

- Issues relating to life and death
- Concerns about the impact of cancer on family and friends
- Treatment procedures and outcomes
- Physical reactions to medical treatment (such as nausea)
- Insurance coverage
- Impaired sexual function
- Financial worries
- Quality of life issues, including concern about finding and maintaining relationships with caregivers
- Family dynamics, including long-lost relatives appearing at the door
- Spiritual issues such as anger at God or feelings of abandonment
- Loss of control
- Loss of friends, because often, even their closest friends do not know how to respond to their needs

The list seems endless—and overwhelming. Cancer patients often find it hard to focus on anything for any length of time. Their "new normal" is a mind that wanders from this to that, from here to there and back again.

Unfortunately, extended visits to the hospital are likely to compound the problem. Consider these environmental and/or psychosocial contributors to attention deficit disorder:

- **Being indoors:** Lack of sunlight reduces melatonin, a key to better sleep.
- **Stress:** Reduced serotonin is believed to be the reason for many cases of mild to moderate depression, which can lead to symptoms such as anxiety, apathy, fear, feelings of worthlessness, insomnia, and fatigue.
- **Lack of exercise:** This results in decreased serotonin and dopamine, the latter of which acts as a powerful regulator of cognitive brain functions.
- **Lack of sleep:** Reduces serotonin.
- **Poor nutrition:** Reduces serotonin.
- **Boredom and lack of activity:** Reduces dopamine and norepinephrine, the latter of which aids the body's response to stress.
- **Deionized air:** Reduces serotonin.[1]

If the above quality-of-life indicators contribute to attention deficit disorder, common sense suggests that an extended stay even in the best hospital will likely compromise a person's ability to concentrate. Few patients get much exercise, sunlight, or sound sleep in a hospital. Boredom and restlessness are common. Most people do not eat well, if for no other reason than they often lose their appetites while at the hospital. And the air? I don't know of anyone who would describe the air in a hospital as refreshing.

Those who suffer from chronic fatigue syndrome (CFIDS) also experience difficulty concentrating. Research shows that in CFIDS patients, fatigue is often accompanied by nonrestorative sleep (95 to 100 percent of patients), confusion combined with an inability to think clearly (75 to 100 percent), and concentration/attention deficit disorder (70 to 100 percent).[2] Therefore both the ADD and CFIDS populations share in some of the same symptoms.

Addressing the importance of hope in the healing equation, author Katrina Berne asked these questions: So how do we "get" hope? How can we maximize and develop it? Her answers virtually all have "focus" as a common denominator. Among others, she suggested,

> Focus on "right now." The Alcoholics Anonymous approach of "one day at a time" can be remarkably helpful.
>
> When we focus on our deprivations, which is natural, we need to be aware of our blessings as well—not either/or but a balance of both. We can learn to appreciate the small stuff—the beauty of sunlight captured in a prism, a child's smile, a funny movie.
>
> Plan something to look forward to. Have short-term goals that are simple and achievable in order to create feelings of accomplishment.[3]

In sum, people who struggle with their ability to concentrate need caregivers around them who will encourage them to focus—to maintain their center.

An electrical high wire carries 10,000 volts of electricity. It enters into a transformer that decelerates the voltage into 110 or 200 volts for common usage in a household. We all have "emotional" transformers. Some of us can take a lot of voltage and maintain our emotional equilibrium. Others can take very little voltage before they are destabilized. However, everyone has a limit as to how much voltage they can take, and when we're hit with a maximum surge of emotional energy, our capacity to think clearly is compromised. Even the thickest-skinned and most emotionally disconnected person has a limit. If the trauma is created by chronic situations or circumstances, such as cancer or other potentially life-threatening diseases, a person's ability to focus is temporarily impaired, and with it their ability to experience joy. This is true for the caregiver as well as the patient.

The stress of caregiving can affect you as well, but my experience is that as difficult as it may be on you the caregiver, it is significantly higher for the patient. If you are having trouble concentrating, imagine what it must be like for the patient.

Although helping your loved one maintain focused concentration may not be easy, there is little you can do that is of greater importance. Consider these words by Og Mandino:

> The weakest living creature, by concentrating his powers on a single object, can accomplish good results while the strongest, by dispersing his effort over many chores, may fail to accomplish anything. Drops of water, by continually falling, hone their passage through the hardest of rocks but the hasty torrent rushes over it with hideous uproar and leaves no trace behind.[4]

Concentrate on what? Focus on what? In the following chapters I'll provide some guidelines that will improve your ability to focus, but the short answer to these questions is *joy*. And the quickest way to the experience of joy is scheduling your time.

An all-too-typical encounter with a cancer patient and caregiver goes as follows: I enter the room. The television is on. Patient is either sleeping or mindlessly staring at the tube. Both the caregiver and patient seem listless and bored. Books are all around, but none are being read. CD players are available, but no music is playing.

I often give them a piece of paper and tell them to write down their schedule; how do they plan on spending their time that day? I encourage them to be as detailed as possible: Schedule your bath, your rest, your breakfast, lunch, and dinner. Schedule your treatments, but don't forget to schedule your Bible study and prayer time. Schedule time to plan your day, even if it is nothing more than reading a *TV Guide* to determine what shows are on the television that you would really want to watch. If you do not plan your time, you are going to waste it.

The following chapters will help you learn about how to experience a quality, joyful life during the brief time we spend in this world. Life is too short to waste our time.

CHAPTER EIGHT

Flow into Joy!

❖

THOUGH THE FIG TREE DOES NOT BUD
AND THERE ARE NO GRAPES ON THE VINES,
THOUGH THE OLIVE CROP FAILS
AND THE FIELDS PRODUCE NO FOOD,
THOUGH THERE ARE NO SHEEP IN THE PEN
AND NO CATTLE IN THE STALLS,
YET I WILL REJOICE IN THE LORD,
I WILL BE JOYFUL IN GOD MY SAVIOR.

—Habakkuk 3:17–18

THE BEST MOMENTS USUALLY OCCUR WHEN A PERSON'S BODY OR MIND IS
STRETCHED TO ITS LIMITS IN A VOLUNTARY EFFORT TO ACCOMPLISH SOMETHING
DIFFICULT AND WORTHWHILE.

—Mihaly Csikszentmihalyi

THE BIBLICAL CONCEPT OF JOY

My life verse is 1 Thessalonians 5:16: "Be joyful always." These words were written by the apostle Paul while in Athens, after he had experienced relentless humiliation, rejection, and persecution. I often tell my patients that if Paul could experience joy in the midst of his difficulties, perhaps we can experience it in a hospital—particularly one filled with optimism, hope, and encouragement. Joy, Paul suggested, should be a constant in our lives and should be especially obvious to others during those times when things are not going the way we would like them to.

Read again the passage from Habakkuk at the beginning of the chapter. Considering the author probably depended on the fertility of his flocks and fields for his livelihood, his situation couldn't have gotten much worse! And yet, even in the midst of his own poverty, he still rejoiced in the Lord.

Joyfulness ought to describe our attitude. As we all know, our truest nature comes out when we are pressed hard. Christians, whose faith has been given its contours by Scripture, ought to be joyful, but often we get depressed instead.

We do well to remember these wise words: "All the darkness in the universe can not extinguish the light of a single candle." Be a candle of hope for your friend.

FROM DEPRESSION TO JOY

As I mentioned in the last chapter, one of the quickest ways to alleviate depression is to regain our focus. But what are we to focus our minds on? What should be the object of our attention? More simply: OK, I agree, but how can I do it? What do I have to do to be happy again? Good question, and one I will answer shortly, but first consider this.

Most cancer patients tell me they are "fine." And I believe they mean it. Here's the problem: For many cancer patients, it has been so long since they have felt happy, they no longer know or remember what "happy" feels like. They are like a fish swimming in a bowl of dirty water. After a while, when you ask the fish how it manages in the dirty water, the fish responds, "What dirt?" In other words, dirty water is its new normal, its new emotional and spiritual baseline.

People are much like that. Many people I see at the cancer hospital are swimming in a bowl of toxic anxiety and negativity; their new normal is summed up in the pronouncement, "I'm fine!" Why? Because they no longer remember what it feels like to be happy and joyful. I have to teach them how to be happy all over again, a necessary step since there's a high correlation between happiness and high immune function. Similarly, there's a high correlation between chronic anxiety and poor immune function. As a professional caregiver to cancer patients, I see too many people swimming in a sea of toxic anger, frustration, and sadness.

If you and/or the patient want to swim away from emotional toxicity, I believe I can help you. To do so, I need to introduce you to a concept called "flow."

Flow as an emotional experience is similar to the biblical experience of joy. Joy isn't emotional ecstasy. It's the feeling deep inside of knowing that, with God's help, the future will be satisfactory, even if it involves pain or the prospect of death. This captures an understanding of joy: In spite of difficulties, one has the ability to praise God with confidence that his love remains.

After all, anyone can be joyful when times are good and there are no dark clouds overhead, but maintaining that attitude while facing a life-threatening challenge—now *that's* the joy displayed by Habakkuk, Paul, Jesus, and his disciples.

As a psychological concept, flow is a source of mental energy that focuses attention and motivates action.[1] We experience flow during long conversations with good friends when the hours that pass seem like minutes. We experience flow when we are totally absorbed in a project we enjoy. We experience flow when we are engaged in an activity and ask ourselves, "Where has the time gone?"

Rarely do people experience flow in passive leisure activities such as watching television or just relaxing.[2] And yet, watching television or listening to music is many patients' primary activity. The problem isn't what they're watching or listening to; the problem is these activities aren't engaging—they're passive and do not require much, if any, interaction.

Flow is the by-product of total concentration and is considered by some psychologists to be a maximum emotional experience and desirable emotional goal. Sports psychologists refer to this phenomenon as being "in the zone." While living in Chicago, I had the opportunity to watch Michael Jordan play basketball. It was a thrill to watch him—he seemed to almost always be in the zone, especially when the game was on the line.

Tiger Woods and other top golfers often find themselves on "hot streaks," when virtually every ball seems to go into the hole. In his book *Golf Is Not a Game of Perfect*, Bob Rotella suggested that the key to "letting it flow" is thinking only about the target. Inside 120 yards, forget about the mechanics of your swing, he said, and concentrate only on putting the ball into the hole.[3]

Of course, this requires maximum concentration and is much easier said than done. But let's not miss the point. Concentration is the key to success not only in the game of golf but also as an influence on our ability to enjoy life.

One expert in the field of flow is Doc Childre, PhD, the founder of the Institute of HeartMath. The Institute of HeartMath has been studying the relationship between our emotions and our physiology or physical well-being. Their studies have revealed clear changes in the patterns of activity of the autonomic nervous system, immune system, hormonal system, brain, and heart when we experience emotions such as appreciation, love, care, and compassion. Dr. Childre is the author of many books on the experience of flow. When asked to explain flow, he said,

> People have talked about "getting in the zone" for years and the zone has become a popular buzzword with dozens of books written on it. But what the "zone" actually is has been hard to pin down, leaving it mysterious and almost unapproachable. Our research has shown that people have within them a place of higher consciousness where life and all kinds of experiences can be processed from another level of intelligence, which we term heart intelligence. It's a

state of heart/brain synchronization that's within all people. There have been many different disciplines to approach it—spiritual and yoga disciplines, breathing, visualization, physical training, etc. These approaches are all akin to each other yet describe different slices of the pie. They all lead to a higher intelligence potential that is within the human capacity to unfold. The zone is not a place—it's a state of consciousness where your higher motor faculties and intuition merge in liquid coordination. You don't just push a button to get there. Entering the zone is an internal developmental process, though people have random heightened experiences of the zone giving confirmation that there is such a state.

Many have experienced times while writing, giving talks, playing music, playing sports, etc., when they felt an intuitive connection with what they were doing and everything flowed. Or days that they moved through their stresses in a liquid way with minimum resistance and energy drain. Or days that flowed with positive synchronicities. These are all aspects of connecting with your heart intelligence rather than a one-shot place of magical peak experience. Then zone achievement becomes more hopeful and the process more simple.[4]

Imagine your life as a caregiver flowing with "positive synchronicities." What if while helping your mother, father, child, or friend, you moved through your stresses "in a liquid way with minimum resistance and energy drain"? Time would fly by, and your worries and fears would give way to smiles, happiness, and a sense of accomplishment as you concentrated on accomplishing an enjoyable task. Worth considering, wouldn't you say?

It is probably difficult for your loved one to experience flow, since concentration is essential to it. Left unattended, minds grow weeds—sadness and self-pity begin to creep in and form a mind that finds it next to impossible to concentrate on anything.

Virtually everyone who has studied the emotional and spiritual phenomenon of flow equates it with deeply spiritual or highly creative experiences. The good news is that anyone who has the ability and willingness to become totally absorbed in a meaningful activity can and will experience flow. Ordinary people like you and me can experience the most positive and healthful feeling of happiness and joy at will if we truly want to.

As the Scriptures teach, "Where your treasure is, there your heart will be also" (Matt. 6:21). Seek to find happiness and joy—first for yourself and then for your loved one.

Helping a cancer patient enter into flow is critically important. As mentioned before, stress degrades immune function. If I as a caregiver can successfully distract a patient from worrying about cancer and the side effects of cancer treatment, I will have enhanced that person's immune function. Further, if I'm able to bring joy into his or her life (which is the primary goal of experiencing flow), I will not only increase immune function I will also have enhanced his or her quality of life.

For someone battling cancer, the experience of flow may be a lifesaver—lengthening the number of days while filling them with meaning and joy. Not a bad experience for those of us helping cancer patients, either.

LIFE WITHOUT FLOW

Let's revisit, for a moment, that depressing outpatient clinic where dozens of people are hooked up to IVs while receiving chemotherapy. The smell is unsettling. Patients are having difficulty coping with their situation. An ever-present "ka-lug, ka-lug" punctuates the silence, reminding everyone of the IV machines as they monitor the distribution of cancer-fighting drugs.

Some of the machines begin to "beep-beep" because the cycle is over or the machine has detected a kink in the plastic tubing. Then there is the tick, tick, tick of the clock on the wall. The tick repeats in a monotonous pattern, yet time seems to stop. Boredom sets in. Conversation, even among good friends, becomes sporadic. And these questions invariably creep into the conversation: How do you feel? Is there anything I can do for you? What can I do to make you feel better?

Would you like some more ice? Have you heard from your family today? Do you feel like going out for a walk? How much longer before the IV is finished? What are you thinking about? Is your faith strong today? How is your attitude? The questions repeat along with well-meaning advice. Don't worry. It's going to be OK. Keep the faith. We're gonna beat this.

And then there's the waiting. Waiting for the drugs to arrive from the pharmacy. Waiting for the nurses to get the drugs. Waiting for the nurses to hook you up. Waiting for lunch. Waiting for the doctors to come by. Waiting for the *Dr. Phil* show to come on. Waiting for the OK to go home. Waiting to hear the lab results. Waiting for e-mail. Sometimes it seems like life is nothing but waiting ... waiting ... waiting. Like waiting for a jury to come back with its verdict. And until it arrives, you feel you are being held in a detention center awaiting your freedom.

What are patients doing while they wait? Perhaps they are engaged in idle chitchat, trying to sleep, reading, or watching television. Do you notice what is missing? Fun! Do you see smiles and hear laughter? No. Are there visible signs of people enjoying life? Obvious manifestations of hope? No. It's business as usual, and right now business isn't very good.

Yet, the business of life is to make every minute count!

Life without flow is manageable. Frankly, many of us go through most of our lives without flow, perhaps because we've never learned how to live any other way. But it's not the best way to experience life.

How many people do you know who experience flow? My guess is that most are living their lives day by day without any clear objectives or focused intention. Perhaps that's why so many people take antidepressants. Unfocused lives are boring! There's no sense of accomplishment, and without experiencing accomplishment unfocused people often develop low self-esteem—a short step away from despair and depression. Like many of us, they are treading water in a lukewarm sea of mediocrity. Or as one good friend puts it, "Dog-paddling on the sea of life." Such is life without flow. The television goes on. Let the surfing begin.

Common sense suggests that if cancer patients have trouble concentrating, the likelihood of their experiencing flow is dramatically reduced. The problem isn't that they can't concentrate—even if they are both able and willing. The problem is most people know little about flow as a preferred experience, much less how to achieve it. They are mentally logjammed, not by choice, but due to a lack of knowing how to free their minds to enjoy life. Given the opportunity, most people would choose to be happy and joyful.

ELEMENTS OF FLOW

Csikszentmihalyi suggests that enjoyment has eight major components. Before you read them, imagine yourself enjoying a favorite activity: scrabble, bridge, tennis, dominoes, crossword puzzles, reading a good book, writing a letter, listening to foot-tapping music. What is it about these experiences that you find enjoyable?

Now consider briefly the eight components of the experience of enjoyment.

1. **The task has a chance of being completed.** Failure to accomplish a goal can be aggravating. By attempting something that's impossible to finish, we emotionally sabotage ourselves and guarantee our experience will be unsatisfying.
2. **Focused attention is given.** Remember the Mental Law of Concentration, which says that a person cannot fully concentrate on two things at one time.
3. **The task has clear goals.** Clarity of rules and goals relieves anxiety and frustration; ambiguity creates stress.
4. **Immediate feedback is provided.** As the pastime activity is engaged, we are not left wondering how we are doing. Frustration is stressful. Instant feedback guarantees that we know if we are playing well or poorly.
5. **Deep and effortless distraction removes worries and frustrations.** Again, it is impossible to be totally absorbed in a pastime and be worried about other things.

6. **Decision-making allows a person to exercise control over his or her actions.** The experience of flow relieves us of the commonly felt burden of powerlessness. As we experience flow, we are empowered to make the best choices possible.
7. **A distraction allows us to lose ourselves in the experience.** Upon finishing the task, we feel stronger and more empowered. Flow allows us to become so fully engrossed in an activity that we intuitively know how the game is played, as well as how it could be played better.
8. **A sense of time is altered.** Flow enables us to transcend our ordinary experience of time and enter into a period of "timeless time."

He adds that "the combination of all of these elements causes a sense of deep enjoyment that is so rewarding people feel that expending a great deal of energy is worthwhile simply to be able to feel it."[5]

Now, compare your enjoyable experience or pastime against this list. Do you see any similarities? As I play Scrabble, I find all of these elements present. I'm forced to concentrate. I know the rules. I know how I am doing by comparing my score to my opponents'. For a while, at least, I'm not worried about life's problems. Time flies by. As I play, I feel happy. If I win, great, but if not, at least I know I played as well as I could.

Imagine, for a moment, a different hospital. This one is filled with patients and medical staff experiencing flow. Do you see that man walking down the hall in his robe while rolling his IV stand loaded with cancer-killing chemicals? Sad, right? Wrong. He's also carrying an iPod and listening to Mozart's Violin Concerto No. 3 or Judy Garland's "Over the Rainbow" or Louis Armstrong's "What a Wonderful World" or Van Morrison's "Brown Eyed Girl" or Linda Ronstadt's "Blue Bayou" or Gloria Gaynor's "I Will Survive" or Selah's version of "It Is Well with My Soul." The bottom line is that his life is qualitatively happier than it would have been had he not tried to make every minute count. And his mind isn't filled with negativity, but good things—very good things.

Now imagine him on his way to an art class where he's learning how to draw or paint. Or to another class where he will learn how to sculpt clay or carve wood or write poetry. Imagine a violinist strolling around the hospital softly playing his instrument. Imagine a patient resting with his family photo album on his lap while writing narratives about the people in the photos. Imagine him engrossed in a cross-word puzzle or Bible study or memorizing his favorite piece of prose, poetry, or Scripture.

These patients' minds are filled with good thoughts. Negativity, stress, and depression are dispelled. The thought of a person who is infirm and yet joyful is jarring and contradictory to many of us. When a person is ill, we imagine just the opposite of joyfulness. Herbert Bensen, MD, a professor at Harvard Medical School, teaches these three truisms to his medical students:

1. **What you believe is what you become.** This teaching parallels Proverbs 23:7 (KJV): "As he thinketh in his heart, so is he." It represents age-old wisdom we ought to take seriously. What do you believe about disease and your loved one's future? If you are thinking negatively, you will be hard-pressed to provide hopeful, helpful caregiving.
2. **What you feel is what you attract.** If a hospital genuinely cares about its patients and their physical, spiritual, and emotional health, it will attract patients who value life and living. In addition, if it genuinely cares about the well-being of the patient's caregivers, this adds a whole new quality to their caregiving network.
3. **What you imagine is what you create.** Too many hospitals have created space filled with unhappiness, sadness, and despair. These spaces are counterproductive to healing. My imagination takes me in a different direction. As a Christian I do not fear death, so don't surround me with sad faces and gloomy spaces. Give me

hope, not pity. Give me a sweet taste of heaven, not the bitterness of hell. Give me love by hugging me, not by keeping a measured, socially acceptable distance. Let me see love and hope in the faces of people at my bedside. Let me feel their sincerity through their willingness to serve me during my greatest hour of need.

One time I was with a parishioner and friend who was very near death. As he lay there with labored breathing, I leaned close to him and said, "Hey, I've got one for you. Wanna hear it?" His eyes gleamed, and he nodded his head. I told my little joke, and he laughed and laughed. It was good. Very good. Just because people are critically ill doesn't mean their spirits can't be lifted or their hope rekindled for one more day.

IT'S ABOUT THE PATIENT

I learned a wonderful lesson from a friend of mine, Gary Fields, a retired superintendent of a nearby school district and a wonderful, capable, and caring man. While comparing the similarities of church management to the complexities of overseeing a large school district, Gary shared that he never had any problem with any teacher whose primary concern was for the children. His mantra was and is "It's about the children." He spoke it often and even had it written on the blackboard in his conference room. It's about the children!

In a hospital, it's about the patient. It's not about the doctors, nurses, chaplains, hospital administrators, or support staff. It's about the patient. We need to continually be asking ourselves how we can help our loved ones find joy in the midst of life's difficulties. In the next chapter, we'll look at ways to help them find joy and flow through pastime management.

CHAPTER NINE

The Art of Pastime Management

The concept of flow is simply about viewing life as a game or pastime, determining what it is about the pastime of life that is enjoyable, and projecting these elements into our daily living. The bottom line, according to Csikszentmihalyi, is how we feel about ourselves and about what happens to us. To improve the quality of life one must improve the quality of experience.[1]

IMPROVE THE QUALITY OF EXPERIENCE

My goal is to improve the quality of your life and the life of your loved one, and I can only do this by improving your experiences—while in the hospital, and then hopefully as you return home. To that end, let's focus on what is perhaps the most important component of the experience of enjoyment: confronting a task that can be completed.

In light of a patient's struggle to concentrate, helping them to identify tasks that have at least the potential to bring joy is, I believe, one of the caregiver's primary tasks. Your ability to do this immeasurably helps the rest of the medical team. The fact that you know your loved one well means that you probably know what he or she might find enjoyable—the "games" the person might like to play.

DOES THE PASTIME STRETCH AND AMUSE YOU?

A key component to flow is engaging in a task that stretches our abilities. If the pastime is something that can be accomplished without thinking, the mind will be easily distracted into dwelling on depressing thoughts, which defeats the whole purpose: relief from suffering. I know women who effortlessly crochet—their hands are busy, but they can carry on a conversation while they crochet. It doesn't stretch them. While their needlework may interest and amuse them, it isn't creating flow, because their minds are easily distracted.

Remember the Mental Law of Concentration: Weeds will grow in our minds unless we intentionally plant flowers (or as author Barbara Johnson put it, "Plant a geranium in your cranium"). Mindless knitting is equivalent to equally mindless channel surfing if you are already an expert knitter. For a beginner, learning how to knit or sew can very easily create flow. Why? Because it stretches you. Learning how to knit is a game that requires full concentration and employs all the necessary characteristics of the experience of enjoyment.

Consider stretching your loved one and yourself in one or more of the following areas.

EXPAND YOUR KNOWLEDGE OF THE BIBLE

There are plenty of online Bible studies with printable questions and answers. There are also hundreds of other Bible study resources available. This would be a wonderful time for you both to grow spiritually while your friend is having physical needs met. If you need guidance, ask your pastor or chaplain to help you identify some material for you to use and/or share with your loved one.

MEMORIZE

Remembering names or favorite Bible passages is a stretch for most of us, and yet when we take the time to memorize anything, we feel a sense of accomplishment. If you want something to enter into your long-term memory, you must commit yourself to repeating it over and over again. Unless you have a photographic memory, there are no shortcuts.

It took me the better part of three hours to memorize 1 Corinthians 13 (the love chapter). The best part is that I can now recite it backward and forward, and it always blesses me to recall it. Get some index cards and carry them around with you. Record your selected passage so you can replay it. Use memory tricks to help you with the memorization process. You can do it! Now would be an excellent time to stretch your mind by memorizing a Bible passage, a poem, a song, or words to your favorite hymn. Quiz each other on what you've memorized—or learn the same songs or Bible passages together.

DO CROSSWORD PUZZLES

If they fall within your ability level, crossword puzzles can be both engaging and fun. If they are too difficult, however, attempting them can be counterproductive, creating stress instead of flow. Occasionally, my wife will start a puzzle and then give the unfinished puzzle to me to see if I can fill in any additional blanks—and vice versa.

WATCH GREAT MOVIES

Some people add that watching funny movies is especially helpful. With regard to flow, any movie that truly entertains you both is what I would recommend. Some hospitals have begun "movie nights" for their patients. Great idea.

PLAY GAMES

Playing games seems an obvious way to pass the time, and yet rarely do I see cancer patients playing Monopoly or chess. Is it because they think they shouldn't have fun? Occasionally I see people playing card games, which, of course, is good. But, again, if the game requires little or no effort to play, then it may be fun, but it's not helping you experience flow.

LEARN TO LAUGH

Scouring the newspaper or Internet for a funny story not only helps create flow, but also a good joke is a gift that keeps on giving. The physical benefits of humor are well known. According to the American Cancer Society,

> Scientists today believe that, even though humor cannot cure disease, it has profound physical and psychological benefits.
>
> As with so many mind-body situations, humor provides relief from worry. In so doing, it relaxes and reduces stress. Endorphins

are released. The entire process is helpful, and it can enhance the quality of life.

Like other complementary therapies, humor therapy may be used in relieving certain symptoms of cancer and side effects of cancer treatment. Humor therapy should not be expected to slow or reverse growth or spread of cancer.[2]

While humor may not "slow or reverse the growth or spread of cancer," even phrasing the statement this way corrupts the mind-set needed for healing. The Bible teaches "believe and you will receive." Remember, "What you believe is what you become." Here's the point: I believe the experience of laughter heals me. It may not cure me, but the experience of laughter, as well as other positive experiences, helps create the best environment for good things to happen.

As poet W. H. Auden put it: "Among those whom I like or admire, I can find no common denominator, but among those whom I love, I can: all of them make me laugh." Another poet, Lord Byron, said it differently: "Always laugh when you can. It is cheap medicine." However, the Bible puts it best: "A cheerful heart is good medicine, but a crushed spirit dries up the bones" (Prov. 17:22). Laugh often. It is good medicine for you.

CREATE AN ETHICAL WILL

Because none of us knows how long we are going to live, we all should have a will that helps dispose of our assets in accordance with our wishes. However, most of us do not think about having an "ethical will," a will that speaks our heart to loved ones by putting our values, our blessings, our deepest thoughts, and remembrances on paper. Barry Baines, MD, has provided a wonderful resource: *Ethical Wills*. He offers several suggestions for starting your own ethical will.[3] Consider exploring these questions with your loved one:

- The lessons I've learned in life are ...
- The event that had the biggest impact on who I have become is ...
- Critical decisions I have made are ...

* What I will miss when I am gone is/are …
* My hopes for the future are …
* What I hope my friends will say about me at my funeral is …

STRETCH YOUR SELF-AWARENESS

Socrates is famously quoted as saying, "An unexamined life is not worth living." Of course, an overly examined life might not be worth living either, but let's not miss the point: Self-examination can produce some helpful results and foster personal peace.

When was the last time you and your loved one learned anything new about yourselves? Take a personality test. Explore with others the implications of what you learn. Dozens of Web sites offer personality tests. Some are free and others are not. After years as the administrator of personality tests (primarily the Myers-Briggs Type Indicator test), I recently took a new and unfamiliar test (the Firo-B test) that helped me better understand my relationships with people who are difficult to get along with.

Learning is a lifelong endeavor. Learn something new about yourself and explore ways in which your strengths have worked for you and your weaknesses have worked against you. Change what you can. Accept what you cannot.

EXPAND YOUR CIRCLE OF FRIENDS

Good friendships grow out of effort and self-disclosure. Making friends takes effort, but getting to know someone can be a very rewarding experience. Get them to tell you their story. Share yours with them. Write them when they go home. Robert Louis Stevenson once said, "A friend is a present you give yourself." Stretch yourselves—make a friend—be a friend.

BE ARTISTIC

Engaging in artistic endeavors is a balm for the soul. Throughout history, art has been used in healing rituals. The ancient Greeks used art effectively to revitalize a patient's inner resources and restore their will to live.[4]

Encourage your loved one to join you in discovering the joy of creating a painting or a drawing. Write a poem or short story. Allow the art, whatever form it might take, to reflect what is going on inside you. Allow it to display your hope, your joy! If you have sadness, get it out by putting it on paper. If you have anger, throw it fiercely onto canvas. If you have grief, give shape to it with clay. If you are feeling spiritually renewed, write a song. If you remember a special feeling you had one time with someone you love, express that feeling in words or images.

Don't worry about whether people like it. It's not for them, anyway. I once saw a painting that was a large red square with a white line down the middle. It was by a modern master, and although the meaning behind much modern art often escapes me, clearly this artist was passionately displaying his inner world. Perhaps the red color symbolized love, and the white line symbolized the boundary line that separated two would-be lovers. Who knows?

According to the American Art Therapy Association, art therapy is based on the belief that the creative process involved in the making of art is healing and life enhancing. Through creating art and talking about art and the process of art making with an art therapist, one can increase awareness of self, cope with symptoms, stress, and traumatic experiences, enhance cognitive abilities, and enjoy the life-affirming pleasures of artistic creativity.[5]

Shands AGH, a community hospital in Gainesville, Florida, has created an extensive Arts in Healing program. It has as part of its staff three artists-in-residence—an oral historian who works with patients to help them tell their stories, an artist who paints small pastel portraits of patients or family members to be given as gifts, and a musician who plays piano and guitar throughout the hospital and serves as a mentor and volunteer coordinator. One patient was quoted as saying, "I didn't know you could have this much fun in a hospital!"[6] Another hospital works with a local clowning group and has "Clowns on Rounds" as part of its volunteer programs. Fun!

Fun is good. Very good. But flow is better, much better, for you and your loved one. I'd rather have you painting than being painted.

I'd rather have you interviewing than being interviewed. I'd rather see you playing music than being played for. I'd rather see you entertaining others through clowning than being entertained. Perhaps the best of both worlds would be to use both aspects by having artists engaging in their art forms as well as encouraging patients and caregivers to explore their own artistic interests.

LEARN A NEW SONG OR SING THE OLD ONES

According to the American Music Therapy Association, the idea of music as a healing influence on illness and behavior is as least as old as the writings of Aristotle and Plato. The twentieth-century discipline began after World War I and World War II when community musicians of all types, both amateur and professional, went to veterans' hospitals around the country to play for the thousands of servicemen suffering both physical and emotional trauma from the wars. The patients' noticeable physical and emotional responses to music led the doctors and nurses to request hospitals to hire musicians.[7]

Nearly everyone has a song that is special to them, that can cause them to forget their worries. My mother-in-law was very feeble and bedridden. I asked her what song floods her with good feelings, and she immediately replied, "Stardust"! Thoughts of Benny Goodman and Glenn Miller filled her heart with such delight. She began to sing, humming the tune when she forgot the words. She might have been bedridden, but in the moment she sang she was sliding on a dance floor with her husband, Miles, who, though deceased, was just as present with her in her heart as ever before.

What is your song? How much effort would it take to explore your loved one's musical tastes? Make a list of songs that can fill his or her heart and mind with joyful, hopeful, and meaningful notes and lyrics.

Significant scientific studies have been conducted on the physiological benefits of music. In his book *The Mozart Effect* Don Campbell relates studies and anecdotal stories about a wide range of diseases, including cancer. One such study focused on certain cancer cells being routinely exposed to the sound of a xylophone. The study reported that "when repeatedly exposed to this sound the nuclear and the cytoplasmic membrane of the cancer cell would break down, its structure thrown into complete disorganization after twenty-one minutes. The healthy cells, however, remained intact."[8]

Again, I am not trying to focus on the healing effects of music, although I do believe music has a soothing and healthful effect. But for the purpose of this book I am more interested in music's ability to create and sustain flow. To that end, music must become a game of sorts. It becomes a game for me when I try to memorize the words to favorite songs. It becomes a game when I search for "oldies" that make me want to shout or sing them out loud. I can get lost in music, but only when I am personally engaged with it. Learning how to play an instrument, if it isn't too stressful, could be an excellent way to creatively enter flow through music.

Here's a suggestion: Bring a CD player to the hospital with a lot of your favorite CDs. Listen to them just for the fun of it. If you're like me, you won't know all of the words. Focus on one song that you want to learn all the words to. Play the song over and over until you find yourself getting lost in the music. Let the music and all the memories attached to it take you far, far away.

ENGAGE YOUR MIND THROUGH READING

Because concentration can be difficult for many people, especially those who face life-threatening diseases, reading can be a struggle. However, the act of reading something enjoyable engages the mind and fulfills all the categories required to experience flow.

Begin with a book's preface or introduction if there is one. It introduces the subject matter and gives context to that which follows. Assuming that you are not in a hurry, try to understand why the author has spent the time and effort writing the book. What is the essence of the book, its core purpose? Does it look like this book is going to be worth your time and effort? Read the first chapter. The purpose of the first chapter is to draw the reader into wanting to read more. If the first chapter doesn't do this for you, chances are the rest of the book isn't going to be any more satisfying.

The mayor of the city of Denver, with great success, selects one book per month and challenges the entire city to read and discuss it. During your loved one's hospital stay, why not get a group of friends or family members together to read and discuss a certain book? Many books (including this one) have discussion guides in the back to help facilitate conversation and enhance enjoyment. As you read, take notes or highlight meaningful passages. As new thoughts enter your mind, write them down or type them into some sort of critical narrative. Resist the temptation to allow your eyes to skim or glaze over the pages. If this is how you read, you might end up with a pile of books that you've "read," but you will not have experienced flow.

Keep a pencil and pad nearby as you read. If you're reading fiction, make notes of the main characters' names and personality traits. Keep track of plot development. As you finish a chapter, use your intuition to anticipate what you think is likely to happen next. The process can be slow, but books can become much more meaningful—and help with flow—when you pore over the text in a deliberate manner.

CREATE YOUR OWN FAMILY PROJECTS

With a little effort you could probably come up with a dozen or more projects that would bring the entire family into flow. One that comes to mind involves family photos and the untold stories behind them. One of my favorite photos was taken in the late afternoon on a California beach right off of Highway 1. I asked a passerby to take the photo so I wouldn't be absent from this scene, which included a group of seals in the background. What the picture didn't show was that moments earlier our daughter, Sara, had been lying on top of one of the sleeping seals. As the saying goes, every picture tells a story. Spend time telling the stories—write your remembrances and share them with your clan.

CHAPTER TEN

A Sacred Time

---❖---

THOSE WHO PLAN WHAT IS GOOD FIND LOVE AND FAITHFULNESS.

—Proverbs 14:22

A s you can see, one of the challenges of caregiving is learning how to help a friend pass time. It is a time management issue, when you get right down to it. How are we going to spend the minutes, hours, and days that are part of our "here and now"?

MANAGE TIME

W e cannot stop our loved one's pain. We cannot cure the disease or predict the future. What we do have some control over is the here and now. If we focus our attention on a pleasurable task, our tendency to focus on our pain is diminished.

Marathon runners can race in inclement weather or push through physiological discomfort by concentrating on their breathing or by using their imagination to take their minds off of their pain.

As a twenty-five-year-old I sprained my ankle while running. It was beginning to swell, and I knew I needed to put ice on it in a hurry. I got a small trash can and filled it with lots of ice and a little water. Anyone who has ever had to endure soaking their foot or hand in ice water for any length of time knows how painful it can be. As my foot entered the water, I lay back on my bed and began to meditate—

I imagined that I was far away, walking on a beach. I could almost feel the breeze on my face and the water lapping at my feet. I couldn't help but notice that my foot, which initially had begun to hurt, suddenly felt like it was soaking in a bucket of warm water. There was no pain at all, and I left my foot in the bucket for fifteen minutes while maintaining my imaginative walk along the beach.

At one level this sounds like self-hypnosis. It is. But don't miss the point. Self-hypnosis is impossible absent the capacity to concentrate. Without the ability to focus my attention on another reality, imagined or not, I wouldn't have been able to keep my foot in the water as long as was necessary.

Recently I asked several senior citizens to share their times of flow. One described an experience her deceased husband had during World War II. Stuck in a foxhole for more than four days in Germany, he was able to endure the fear by concentrating on tunes he had learned as a young man. In his mind, he sang these songs over and over, which helped him cope with his fear, worry, and concern.

Your friend is in a foxhole, of sorts, surrounded by an enemy that wants to destroy him or her. Your job, and mine, is to help the person keep his or her wits, to encourage, to offer reasons for hope, and to plant flowers of joy and optimism so God will be able to effectively heal your friend through the wide means of grace made available to all of us.

FLOW AS THE EXPERIENCE OF SACRED TIME

A life lived with flow is a life filled with purpose, meaning, direction, and accomplishment. It must be much of what life is like in heaven—eternity that is filled not only with joy, but also with time-lessness. I can't imagine sitting around in heaven watching the clock tick its seconds, minutes, and hours. Sounds more like hell to me. Flow is what is lacking in so many lives, and it might well be a reason why existence on earth seems a living hell for so many.

In my years of ministry I have become used to two things: Some people think Sunday worship service (usually they mean the sermon) is too long. Others say they never even look at their watch—that time flies by and they couldn't care less how long the service was. What do you suppose is the difference?

Joseph Martos, in his book *Doors to the Sacred*, speaks of sacred time as "timeless time."

> On certain occasions our consciousness of time is altered and we enter a special time, a sacred moment. Sometimes it is longed for, like the moment our child is born; sometimes the moment is dreaded, like the moment our parent dies. But when the moment arrives it feels different. And it lingers; it does not pass.[1]

Sacred time is also experienced when we reflect on past experiences. Pick up your family album and look at the pictures. Some you will quickly glance over, and others will cause you to linger. And as you do, you may find yourself stepping back in time. That time becomes the present as you remember details about the situation. You relive the moment again as though it was happening now. This is flow.

Miles separate my wife and me from our two daughters, Sara and Becca, and our new granddaughters, Lilly and Molly. However, the screen saver on my computer is a picture of Lilly I took several months ago. As I gaze at her picture, I remember how I arranged for a toy with a small mirror to be placed near her head so that the picture would be not only of her face but also the side of her head, so that I could see her soft ears and neck and beautiful hair. Even describing it to you has made me stop typing to remember the moment. It's almost like I am touching her now. I am surrounded by pictures of Sara and Becca. My home is filled with them, so that even though they are not physically with me, they are here in some intangible, but no less real, way.

Sacred time is time that flows. One of the challenges caregivers have is helping our loved ones pass the time. We cannot always make time go quickly. Life is often lived in ordinary time, but it is helpful to know there are experiences to be enjoyed and that we are not doomed or limited to experience ordinary time. To the extent we can help time pass quickly—and experience timeless time—we can lift our loved one's spirits and keep him or her from thinking about things that cause despair.

DISTRACTIONS: THE ENEMY OF FLOW

The other day I was deep in thought as I was writing the first draft of this book. I don't remember exactly what I was writing about, but I was flowing, effortlessly typing away. Suddenly—and unexpectedly—our handyman entered my study to repair some doorknobs (we've been remodeling an old Victorian home). He didn't speak to me, since it was obvious I was busy writing. Nevertheless he was working five feet from me. I began to stare at the computer. No words were typed. No coherent thoughts or ideas could be conveyed. My concentration had been broken and with it my ability to flow.

Distractions are the nemesis of concentration.

As you help your loved one cope with his or her disease, and as you help the person learn to pass the time by engaging in activities that enable him or her to concentrate on something enjoyable, you learn that life is filled with distractions. Some can be easily dismissed, while others require your full attention. You will know what is required by the circumstances. Occasionally, even when I'm writing, I'll finish a paragraph and not know what to write about next. The flow is gone, and it's time to rest or attempt another task.

Certainly there are times when it is impossible to focus, such as when you are just too tired to care. Give yourself permission to lose your focus from time to time—but not indefinitely.

A wonderful source of flow is meditation or contemplative prayer. Although I am far from an expert in the field of meditation, over the years I have made the effort to develop a contemplative prayer life. The great challenge of contemplative prayer is to focus on a word or pictorial scene—and nothing else. One particular prayer is commonly called "The Jesus Prayer," based on a paraphrase of Matthew 20:31: *Lord Jesus Christ, Son of God, have mercy on me, a sinner.* You might find meditating on this phrase to be fruitful. Often, during moments of deep meditation, timeless time is experienced. Not sleep, but an altered reality where one can hear, smell, and feel, and yet twenty minutes seems like two.

People who are advanced, practiced contemplatives are able to remain in that state of mind for extended periods of time. They can do this because they have mastered the ability to dismiss distracting thoughts. As a thought creeps in, they allow it to pass through their mind, without focusing on it. Some dismiss it by simply saying, "Oh well."

Perhaps your challenge (and mine) is to develop the capacity to flow during the good times as well as during troubled times. Perhaps what you need is a plan that includes an identifiable goal or target that will help you define success as a parent, confidante, child, or friend to the one God has placed into your care.

If the research by the Institute of HeartMath and others is accurate, as reflected by my own experience of Christian joy, you and your loved one will feel better and enjoy an enhanced immune function as well as other biological benefits. Perhaps one of the greatest benefits is experiencing an uplifted spirit at a time of life when the unbelieving world would be filled with despair and sadness.

Plan your day. Make God part of your plan.

> Each day is a special gift from God, and while life may not always
> be fair, you must never allow the pains, hurdles, and handicaps of
> the moment to poison your attitude and plans for yourself and your
> future. You can never win when you wear the ugly cloak of self-pity,
> and the sour sound of whining will certainly frighten away any
> opportunity for success. Never again. There is a better way.[2]
> —OG MANDINO

CHAPTER ELEVEN

Boundaries in Caregiving

A boundary is that invisible moral line in the sand beyond which a person will not go. We all have them. For example, one of my boundaries is my refusal to pity someone with cancer or any other chronic disease. I have a choice: to instill hope or give pity. I prefer to instill hope. That's why I do things some people think are a little strange. For example, our hospital has a waiting room outside our medical clinic, the place where people are waiting to have their blood drawn, medical histories taken, and visit with the medical oncologist.

Often the waiting room, filled with cancer patients and their caregivers, is sad and gloomy. Some people may be in wheelchairs; others have oxygen tanks they are connected to; some are there for the first time and are very frightened. When I see this psychodynamic taking place in the clinic, I often return to my office and pull some karaoke DVDs off my shelf and return to the clinic saying, "Hey, everyone! Anyone feel like singing! Come on, let's go!" And I gather a handful of patients and caregivers around the large, flat-screen TV in the clinic, plug in a DVD, and lead the group in singing songs such as "Take Me Home, Country Roads," "Blue Bayou," or "He Ain't Heavy, He's My Brother." Before long, we have quite a songfest going! And the atmosphere changes … dramatically. Sometimes it takes such little effort to lift people's spirits, and singing familiar songs is usually a surefire way to do it. It takes effort to be happy. If my patients are going to be sad, it is not going to be because I didn't try to help them be happy, even while they are waiting to see a doctor in a cancer hospital. I refuse to let their sadness affect me. Remember: Hope! Not pity! I have my boundaries. And you do too.

The great challenge in caring for others is to help them make decisions that *they* believe are in their best interest, not what you think is in their interest. The goal is to empower your loved one to assume control of and responsibility for their own health care, as long as they don't endanger their life or the lives of others. Nowhere is patient empowerment more important than the decision to execute an advance directive, or living will. The federal government, as well as every state, has laws that require the patient to be made aware of their rights as patients, particularly as they relate to situations when patients, due to their medical condition, are unable to make health-care decisions on their own. An advance directive is the document made available by the state, if not the hospital, that allows patients the opportunity to clearly state their wishes should they reach the point where they are unable to make decisions on their own. Patients are not required to execute the document, but the hospital is required to make patients aware of their rights. What should your role be as a caregiver?

God is pro-life. Even a cursory reading of the Scriptures teaches us that God created life, sustains life, gives life, and takes it away. When it comes to end-of-life decisions, I would offer this suggestion: The two most intimate moments we will ever experience with God are at the moment of new birth (when we give our life to God) and the time God calls us home to him. Both are intensely personal, and I would encourage you to resist the temptation to give undue influence in the decision-making process regarding advance directives. Here's why: As much as we might want our loved one to live, he or she may sense that the time is drawing near. Further, late-stage cancer patients often experience great pain and suffering, together with either tremendous weight loss or swelling, yellowing of skin, and days and days of entering into and out of consciousness. When at last the heart stops, attempts at cardiopulmonary resuscitation often result in breaking the patient's ribs, along with other invasive measures. If this is truly what the patient wants, the health-care team will dutifully oblige. Be aware of your moral boundaries and tremendous influence on the patient: Let your friend be the one to decide what he or she wants. Commit yourself to patient empowerment from beginning to end.

At our hospital, we embrace the concept of Patient Empowerment Medicine. This is what it means to us:

> Patient Empowerment Medicine (PEM) is a philosophy of care that puts patients first and in the center of their care. Aside from assembling a team of expert care providers who work within your schedule (and not the other way around), CTCA works diligently to uncover the things that patients need and value—long before they even enter our doors.[1]

Patient-centered care is a difficult concept for some people to understand. Consider exploring some of these Web sites that will help you become familiar with this concept of medical treatment:

- http://www.patientpower.info/default.asp
- http://www.cancersupportivecare.com/empower.html

I am simply attempting to help you understand that your role as a caregiver is to help your loved one make informed decisions about his or her own health care. Quite bluntly, it is your friend's life, not yours. And to the extent he or she is mentally capable of making rational decisions without causing harm to him- or herself or others, then he or she should be encouraged to do so. The goal is patient empowerment.

Whether I am working with cancer patients or children, I am very aware of my limitations as a caregiver. I cannot make my children love and respect me. I cannot make them eat their vegetables. I cannot force them to do their homework or come home at an agreed-upon hour. What I can do is make my children aware of my love and respect for them. I can treat them as responsible individuals who are worthy of my trust and who are capable of making good choices if given the options and made aware of the alternatives and logical consequences of their decisions.

I am not naive. I know children can and often do make poor choices. But how are they ever going to learn to be responsible individuals if they are not allowed to make choices, if I always make their decisions for them? Clearly, I could try to do that, but what I would end up with is irresponsible, codependent children who are either incapable or unwilling to make difficult choices in their lives. Why? Because someone had always made their choices for them!

A good parent allows his or her children to make decisions, unless they are going to hurt himself or herself or someone else. A good parent would not let a child run into the street, play with matches, or get away with hitting a brother or sister or pulling a pet's tail.

DO NO HARM

There are boundaries with parenting, but there are also boundaries for good caregiving. Good caregivers should try to prevent their loved ones from causing harm to themselves or others. We want our loved ones to assume control over their decisions, and we want to empower them to make decisions with respect to their quality of life. However, we must try to keep them from hurting themselves.

I know of a woman who has repeatedly asked her daughter to aid her in committing suicide. I know of another who continuously asks her caregiver to overmedicate her. Many cancer patients lose their appetites, and some die from malnutrition instead of the cancer itself. Allowing our loved ones to refuse to eat is no different than denying them properly prescribed medication. Although we cannot force-feed them, we can make them aware of the consequences of their decision and let them know how we are hurt by their refusal to allow us to provide proper care.

As Hippocrates taught, and as our doctors so pledge, we as care-givers ought to feel equally committed to fulfilling this teaching by making this motto our own:

> Declare the past, diagnose the present,
> foretell the future; practice these acts.
> As to diseases, make a habit of two things—to help,
> or at least to do no harm.

Even as physicians operate under the credo "Do no harm," so too are we caregivers obligated to care for others under the humane precept of preventing harm—self-inflicted or otherwise.

Remember, you cannot give insights to unmotivated people. Write it upon your heart, your bedpost, or your bathroom mirror. It may be the only bit of advice that keeps you sane. You are limited in your ability to help.

Doctors know this too. As important as the will to live is, the best doctors in the world can't make someone want to live, take medicine, or trust in them or in God. They can't force patients to surround themselves with a system of social support. They can't make them think positive thoughts. Remember this. And pray that your loved one finds the motivation to make rational, positive decisions.

Robert Frost, in his poem *The Road Not Taken*, described many of us:

> Two roads diverged in a yellow wood,
> And sorry I could not travel both
> And be one traveler, long I stood
> And looked down one as far as I could
> To where it bent in the undergrowth;
> Then took the other, as just as fair,
> And having perhaps the better claim,
> Because it was grassy and wanted wear;
> Though as for that the passing there

Had worn them really about the same,
And both that morning equally lay
In leaves no step had trodden black.
Oh, I kept the first for another day!
Yet knowing how way leads on to way,
I doubted if I should ever come back.
I shall be telling this with a sigh
somewhere ages and ages hence:
Two roads diverged in a wood, and I—
I took the one less traveled by,
and that has made all the difference.

What if the road "less traveled by" was the road of joy? Too many of us are so overwhelmed by stress and anxiety, worries and concerns that comprise much of our cultural success-driven ethos, that we do not take the less-traveled road of simplicity, peace, harmony, and joy. The result? We become unbalanced. We do not feel well. We get sick.

Take the time to find joy and peace. It will make all the difference in your life—and the life of your loved one.

Joy has nothing to do with material things,
or with a man's outward circumstances....
A man living in the lap of luxury can be wretched,
and a man in the depths of poverty can overflow with joy.[2]
—WILLIAM BARCLAY

Appreciating Our Way into Better Health

I f life were a musical score, moments of flow or the experience of sacred time would be the notes, and the space between the notes would be ordinary time. We strive to maintain optimum emotional experiences, but we all know that eventually we drift back to reality. Worship eventually ends, and we walk out of the church into the real world. We long for the heightened and satisfying experience of heaven, but we are forced to live most of our lives between the notes—paying bills, buying groceries, and filling the car with gas.

So what can we do to reduce the space between the notes? The focus of this chapter is to help caregivers maintain mindfulness, to help you learn how to recapture joy even in those times that are common and ordinary.

INTENTIONALLY CREATE FEELINGS OF CARE AND COMPASSION

If we were able to intentionally generate "feelings of care and compassion" would we be able to experience higher immune function? The research seems clear: yes.

The Institute of HeartMath has engaged in revolutionary research in the field of neurocardiology. Their research suggests that our emotions are not completely controlled by our brains as has been historically believed, and that the heart itself plays a particularly important role in the emotional system.

In a publication titled *The Appreciative Heart*, researchers Rollin McCraty and Doc Childre suggest that even as we possess a "cranial brain," we also have a "heart brain," which creates and processes emotions far more rapidly than our minds can calculate or respond to. They believe that "with each beat, the heart not only pumps blood, but also continually transmits dynamic patterns of neurological, hormonal, pressure, and electromagnetic information to the brain and throughout the body."[1]

The Institute of HeartMath is dedicated to helping people experience flow, which it calls "coherence." The definition of coherence, as understood within the field of physics, is the ordered and constructive distribution of power within a wave. The more stable the frequency and shape of the waveform, the higher the coherence. Key to understanding this concept is this: Our hearts can be measured for coherence since they produce electromagnetic waves. To the extent that these waves can be directly controlled, a person has the opportunity to choose to enter into this heightened state of flow or coherence.

Further, our hearts not only create wave rhythms, they can also be monitored for resonance, or large vibrations produced in response to various stimuli. According to HeartMath's research, when a heart is in physiological coherence, it produces a peak resonance of around 0.1 hertz, which is the equivalent to a ten-second rhythm. Peak resonance and physiological coherence are highly correlated with times when people are actively feeling appreciation or some other positive feeling.

In other words, to the extent we are able to generate positive feelings (joy, happiness, love, forgiveness, and so forth), we substantially enhance the likelihood of entering into the state of coherence or flow.[2]

The problem is that most of us do not know how to experience these positive feelings at will. Our experience of joy, peace, patience, kindness, and self-control (as well as other feelings) is often spontaneous and sporadic; the notes are often far apart, leaving us with long periods of joyless silence. Studies correlate positive feelings with improved health, increased longevity, enhanced cognitive function including the capacity to focus and pay attention, and a "notable reduction in inner mental dialogue," or reduced negative self-talk.[3]

WALK WITH APPRECIATION

Consider for a moment that your feelings are companions, acquaintances you choose to take a walk with. Perhaps it will be a short walk. Maybe a long, long walk. But the point is that you choose your companions; they do not choose you. You can freely, at will, select to walk with the companion of your choice.

You can choose, for example, to walk with Anger. If you do, you will do the things angry people do. You will be resentful, vindictive, and seek to respond to your problems with a vengeful attitude. Walk with Anger long enough and it'll ruin your life. Anger is a poor companion for those who are fighting disease and will probably ensure a longer recovery period.

A close associate of Anger is Fear. When you choose to walk with Fear, it is impossible to be hopeful and optimistic. Why? Because for every reason Hope and Optimism give you, Fear comes up with a dozen or more reasons why they are wrong. Fear is negative by nature. Fear of death causes a heightened state of anxiety. You can walk with Fear, if you like, but don't expect Fear to lead you to a place of peace. Follow Fear long enough and you will find yourself in the depths of personal agony. Perhaps that is why the Scriptures teach us that "There is no fear in love. But perfect love drives out fear, because fear has to do with punishment. The one who fears is not made perfect in love" (1 John 4:18).

Walk with Fear and you walk away from Love. If you choose to walk with Love, on the other hand, you quickly learn that Love is complex, a multifaceted virtue. The apostle Paul taught that Love is patient and kind, along with many other attributes. However, Paul did not exhaust the definitions of Love nor did he completely unfold all the nuances that determine the qualities of Love.

Modern research has discovered the aspect of Love that is easiest to enter into is the feeling of Appreciation. According to one expert, "Appreciation is the purest, strongest form of love."[4] When we think appreciative thoughts, our normal world stops and a state of grace begins. During active appreciation, your brain, heart, and endocrine system work in synchrony and heal in harmony.[5]

To test this theory, I hooked myself up to a heart monitor. It measured both my heart rate and my heart rhythm using a software program developed by the Institute of HeartMath, a computer program that teaches individuals how to enter into flow at will.

On several occasions I've been angry at someone for doing something that irritated me—typical daily bumps and clashes with friends and family. As I began the computer session, I noticed I was out of flow; my heart rhythms reflected my inner world of anger, producing jagged, distorted lines. I began to think about how much I appreciated the individual who had made me angry. I could think of many things I liked about him—his sense of humor, his willingness to be my friend, the care and concern he and his wife had shown over the years for my family and me. Suddenly my heart rhythm displayed a pattern conducive to a high state of flow—my anger was replaced, at will and in an instant, by appreciation and the ancillary health benefits that attend feeling happy and joyful.

Walk with Appreciation, and you will be free to live instead of bound to suffer.

EXPRESS YOUR APPRECIATION

If stretching ourselves is one of the primary characteristics of entering into an optimum emotional experience, shouldn't we take advantage of the research that suggests we can discover enormous benefits for our hearts and immune system? All it requires is a minute or so in which we focus on something or someone we appreciate or care about. As you enter and leave the hospital, aren't there ample opportunities and numerous reasons to truly appreciate the incredible health-care system God has provided for your loved one?

Years ago, while on a medical mission trip to Ecuador, I was in an operating room where a young surgeon from Texarkana, Texas, was lovingly (and at his own expense) performing surgery on a baby born with a clubfoot. I'll never forget looking up and seeing cobwebs on a ceiling fan. Across the hall were several pregnant women leaning naked against a wall in an attempt to induce labor. The medical clinics in the barrios often had nothing more than aspirin to offer those who had walked miles to be seen by an American doctor. Many of the complaints stemmed from kidney ailments. Why? Because the locals didn't have clean water to drink. When we left, we were all saddened by the hundreds of people standing outside the clinic tearfully waving good-bye to the American doctors, nurses, and support staff.

I have a dear friend who pastors a church in Ghana. Whenever he returns from a visit here he is flooded with people in need of his prayers for healing, in part because Ghanaians do not have the public health benefits that we have come to enjoy and take for granted.

We all owe our very lives to the men and women who have dedicated themselves to healing, and I would encourage you to consider, as a way to relieve your stress, spending several minutes a day focusing your thoughts on the marvelous caregivers all around you who are dedicated to seeing your loved one healed.

The song "Angels Among Us" includes some inspiring lyrics:

Oh I believe there are angels among us....

They wear so many faces,
show up in the strangest places.
To guide us with their mercy, in our time of need.

This song reminds me of Hebrews 13:2, which states, "Do not forget to entertain strangers, for by so doing some people have entertained angels without knowing it."

Angels are often romanticized or portrayed in humorous ways in books and movies. (Remember the comical angel, Clarence, in the classic holiday movie *It's a Wonderful Life?*) Yet angels aren't people who have died and then changed into their new, heavenly form. Angels, according to the Bible, are an entirely different created order of celestial beings whose primary purpose is to praise God and communicate his messages to the rest of us. Doctors and nurses aren't literal "angels," but they are as close as most of us will ever see. Find ways to show your appreciation to the hospital staff.

Whether you find a tangible way to express your appreciation, take advantage of those one-minute Freeze-Frame exercises mentioned in chapter 6 to think about and be thankful for other members of the caregiving team—the doctors, nurses, aides, and other support staff. You might be surprised to learn how much they appreciate you as well. One of the unwritten but much-talked-about goals of the hospital where I work is expressing appreciation—to you as a caregiver, to your loved one, to other staff members, and department heads. Hospitals are like families; we work together, but we also share our lives with one another.

Appreciation is expressed in many ways and is part of our corporate culture. Not because it is good for our health, although that is a wonderful ancillary benefit, but because we all recognize how dependent we are on one another to perform our duties to their fullest.

A patient's fortitude and fighting spirit are marvelous qualities. The resiliency of the human spirit is amazing to behold as difficulties are repeatedly faced and overcome. The dignity many patients exhibit at the end of their life is both moving and exemplary.

Are you still looking for something to appreciate? Look at the wrinkles on any person's face and appreciate the many miles that person has traveled, the pain and joy he or she has experienced along the way. Ask yourself, "What or who caused the wrinkles? Was it me?" Focus on one gray hair on a friend's head and imagine what might have caused it to turn gray, and how this friend has "kept on keepin' on."

And the next time you see a doctor, consider the years of study medical professionals endure en route to that degree. Imagine the long hours of reading and memorizing, the missed sleep, the gallons of coffee required to stay alert, and the sacrificial commitment to helping others that sometimes took them away from family birthday parties and picnics to serve or treat a patient. Admire their pain—the sadness and disappointment felt when they've lost a patient. Say a prayer for them. Ask God to bless them in their ministry to others.

The last place on earth anyone should find it difficult to feel appreciation and caring is in a hospital in the United States of America. From highly advanced medical technology, to highly trained health-care professionals, to extraordinary research facilities, and, of course, to God for providing all of it for us, we have so much to appreciate and care about!

One of my favorite pieces of prose is this beautiful and thoughtful statement by Theodore Roosevelt commonly titled *The Man in the Arena*:

> It is not the critic who counts: not the man who points out how the strong man stumbles, or where the doer of deeds could have done better. The credit belongs to the man who is actually in the arena, whose face is marred by dust and sweat and blood, who strives valiantly, who errs and comes up short again and again, ... who

knows the great enthusiasms, the great devotions, who spends himself for a worthy cause; who, at the best, knows, in the end, the triumph of high achievement, and who, at the worst, if he fails, at least fails while daring greatly, so that his place shall never be with those cold and timid souls who knew neither victory nor defeat.[6]

There isn't a doctor, nurse, administrator, nutritionist, or any other member of the hospital team, including you as a caregiver, who will find his or her "place with those cold and timid souls who knew neither victory nor defeat." We are all "in the arena." Our faces are marred by dust, sweat, and blood. Do we occasionally "come up short again and again"? Of course, and we want to know from you how, so we can make our best efforts better. Yet we must resist the temptation to reduce our observations of health-care professionals to criticisms and harsh judgments. We are all human beings worthy of dignity and respect.

As philosopher Ludwig Wittgenstein once put it, "The world of those who are happy is different from the world of those who are not."[7] The world of those who appreciate and care for others is a different world as well. I invite you to join it—enter into it fully—to appreciate more fully this amazing life we have the opportunity to live, and to care for the world and every person in it as though we all truly were members of the same family.

I leave you now with a great personal sense of hopefulness that some who read this book might actually employ some of my suggestions. Cancer patients have much to teach us, and perhaps the greatest lesson is this: Life is short. Make the most of every minute by living for today. Make a game out of life by making a game out of today.

On the wall of our little hospital chapel hangs a copy of the "Serenity Prayer." It was embroidered by one of our patients, L. M., who, after learning about the benefits of flow, went home and created the lovely wall hanging. Most know of only the first few sentences. The last few, in my view, are the best.

My dear cancer caregiver, may God give you and your loved one serenity as you shine the light of your hope-filled candle into whatever darkness the future may bring. Remember these ancient words: "All the darkness in the universe can not extinguish the light of a single candle."

THE SERENITY PRAYER

God grant me the serenity
to accept the things I cannot change;
courage to change the things I can;
and wisdom to know the difference.
Living one day at a time;
Enjoying one moment at a time;
Accepting hardships as the pathway to peace;
Taking, as He did, this sinful world
as it is, not as I would have it;
Trusting that He will make all things right
if I surrender to His Will;
That I may be reasonably happy in this life
and supremely happy with Him
Forever in the next.
Amen.

—REINHOLD NIEBUHR

Doing All We Can Do—with God's Help

One of the great ironies of my life is that during the writing of this book, I have been undergoing a number of life-changing circumstances, all of which are stressful. When they all come at one time, well, it's pretty tough. Within just a few weeks,

- My two daughters moved far away due to vocational decisions. Very sad.
- I accepted a new position as the director for pastoral care at the Cancer Treatment Centers of America's new hospital, Eastern Regional Medical Center in Philadelphia, and will be moving there soon. Career changes are always stressful.
- I sold a home that I spent an entire year remodeling and had grown to love. The joy of occupying it, at long last, is coming to an end. It's like leaving behind a good friend.
- I'm leaving a parish ministry for the first time in fifteen years and beginning a whole new career, as well as leaving behind many dear friends in my church I have grown to love. The grief is profound.
- My personal life is experiencing the volcanic tremors of midlife, complete with all of the fears and wonders that accompany the realization and acceptance of both my humanity and mortality.

I am imagining a great future for myself. A hopeful series of "coming attractions" is playing out in my heart and mind. But I haven't discovered a silver bullet that inoculates me from sadness, anger, frustration, guilt, sleeplessness, and fear. What I have to offer you in this book is not a silver bullet for you either, but rather a way to effectively cope with life's daily stresses and strains.

I know that in light of the overwhelming stress I am experiencing right now, my immune system is taking a beating. I occasionally feel my heart in a viselike grip and my mind often wanders. My "get it" factor is very high right now when it comes to trying to cope during a time of personal turmoil, and I am even more aware of how difficult it is to maintain focused attention. Having said that, I want to share some personal thoughts about how I am using much of what I have shared in this book.

BIG GOD—LOW HURDLES

God is in control, and it is arrogant to think otherwise. I have hurdles in front of me, and they are many, but they are low hurdles that I will get over with God's help. Time and again God will help me over the obstacles that await me, which, in turn, will help me to remain calm and confident that I will complete the race he has called me to run. The Scriptures teach that "in all things God works for the good of those who love him, who have been called according to his purpose" (Rom. 8:28). All things. Not some things. My God is a big God, and the high hurdles before me are made low by him.

FLOW IS POSSIBLE

I have learned that it is possible to shorten the space between the notes, that the concept of flow can be experienced, and that the relief it promises is real. For example,

- I try a little harder to stay focused by organizing my time better.
- I am writing a personal journal to probe my thoughts and feelings.
- I am watching great movies that take my mind off my problems.
- I am taking my vitamins and eating lots of vegetables with deep and bright colors—the ones with the highest concentration of antioxidants.
- I am exercising more regularly.

- I am entering into the world of music more intentionally and finding my spirits lifted.
- I am spending time engaging in in-depth conversations and discovering moments of timeless time.
- I am seeking the social support of friends.
- I am becoming reinvigorated by taking care of little details around the house that have been disregarded.
- I am training myself to take frequent Freeze-Frame moments and quiet my heart by concentrating on people I care a lot about, their qualities and quirky idiosyncrasies that have enhanced my life over the years.
- I often think of moments that I have cared for others, which help me as much as anything flow into joy.

When I do these things, I feel much, much better. The stress evaporates, and I am confident my ability to cope with life's problems is allowing my immune system to operate at a high level. With God's help, I've done all I can to help myself live a full and abundant life. If today is the day that God calls me home, my heart is at peace.

What I have to offer you is not just a theory to be explored, but also a lifestyle to be lived. And so, my caring friend, as you live and learn and care and serve, take good care of yourself. Really good care.

Let your candle of hope shine brightly. The world needs more people like you.

To the world you might be one person,
but to one person you might be the world.
—UNKNOWN

About the Author

Michael S. Barry is a former pastor and current Director for Pastoral Care at the Cancer Treatment Centers of America at Eastern Regional Medical Center in Philadelphia. He is also the author of the popular books *A Reason for Hope: Gaining Strength for Your Fight Against Cancer* (Life Journey) and *A Season for Hope: Daily Encouragement for Your Fight Against Cancer* (Honor Books).

NOTES

INTRODUCTION: OPENING THE DOOR

1. Susan B. Frampton, Laura Gilpin, and Patrick A. Charmel, eds., *Putting Patients First* (San Francisco: Jossey-Bass, 2003), 52.
2. Michael Moncur, The Quotations Page, http://www.quotationspage.com/quotes/Helen_Keller/ (accessed February 1, 2007).

CHAPTER 1: A PRIVILEGE AND A CHALLENGE

1. Answers Corporation, Answers.com, http://www.answers.com/topic/rip-current (accessed February 1, 2007).
2. Dan Baker and Cameron Stauth, *What Happy People Know* (Emmaus, PA: Rodale, 2003), 92, 94.
3. Stephen C. Lundin, Harry Paul, and John Christensen, *Fish!* (New York: Hyperion, 2000), 31.
4. ThinkExist Quotations, http://en.thinkexist.com/quotes/with/keyword/constitution/ (accessed February 1, 2007).
5. Often I use the words *happiness* and *joy* interchangeably because the feelings we experience as happiness and joy are very nearly identical. However, there are qualitative differences. Happiness, for example, can be found in eating a piece of chocolate cake. Joy? Joy may be found in the healthful decision to let it go.
6. BestMotivation.com, http://www.bestmotivation.com/byauthor/james_allen.htm (accessed February 1, 2007).
7. ThinkExist.com Quotations, http://en.thinkexist.com/quotations/marriage/ (accessed February 1, 2007).
8. Doc Childre and Bruce Cryer, *From Chaos to Coherence* (Boulder Creek, CA: HeartMath, 2000), 63.
9. Galatians 5:22.

CHAPTER 2: PRINCIPLES OF CAREGIVING

1. Barbara Schmidt, Twainquotes.com, http://www.twainquotes.com/Lightning.html (accessed February 1, 2007).
2. Edwin H. Friedman, *Friedman's Fables* (New York: Guilford Press, 1990), 75ff.
3. Martha Heineman Pieper, PhD, and William J. Pieper, MD, *Addicted to Unhappiness* (New York: McGraw-Hill, 2003), 93.
4. Baker and Stauth, *What Happy People Know*, 89.
5. Ibid., 32.
6. HeartMath LLC, HeartQuotes, http://www.heartquotes.net/Health.html (accessed February 1, 2007).

CHAPTER 3: THE MENTAL LAWS OF TRANSFORMATION

1. Brian Tracy, *Maximum Achievement* (New York: Simon and Schuster, 1993).
2. Ibid., 92.
3. Jennifer Cawthorne, "Healing Words." *The Aquarian* (Fall 1999), http://www.aquarianonline.com/Wellness/HealingWords.html (accessed February 1, 2007).
4. Frank Lynch, The Samuel Johnson Sound Bite Page, http://www.samueljohnson.com/persever.html (accessed February 1, 2007).
5. Moncur, The Quotations Page, http://www.quotationspage.com/quotes/Cicero/31 (accessed February 1, 2007).
6. S. E. Locke, et al., "Life Change Stress, Psychiatric Symptoms, and Natural Killer Cell Activity," *Psychosomatic Medicine* 46 (1984): 441–53.

CHAPTER 4: BELIEVING IN GREAT POSSIBILITIES

1. Toastmasters, Quotations Plus+, http://www.oktm.ca/Quotes_content-S.htm (accessed February 1, 2007).
2. Lundin, Paul, and Christensen, *Fish!*, 51.

CHAPTER 5: THE ROLES WE PLAY

1. Patrick Quillen (cancer-seminar lecture, Flint, MI).
2. http://www1.agric.gov.ab.ca/$department/deptdocs.nsf/all/bmi10685.
3. WorldofQuotes.com, http://www.worldofquotes.com/author/Allan-K.-Chalmers/1/index.html (accessed February 1, 2007).
4. HeartMath LLC, HeartQuotes, http://www.heartquotes.net/Happiness.html (accessed February 1, 2007).
5. Lundin, Paul, and Christensen, *Fish!*, 44.
6. Gratefulness.org, "Faith" © 1990 David Whyte, http://www.gratefulness.org/poetry/Faith.htm (accessed February 15, 2007).
7. E. Cameron and L. Pauling, Chem. Bio. Interactions, Vol. 9, p. 272, 1974

CHAPTER 6: BE A REAL FRIEND

1. Victor Frankl, *Man's Search for Meaning* (Boston: Beacon Press, 2006), 66.
2. Baker and Stauth, *What Happy People Know*, 131.
3. http://www.merckmedicus.com/pp/us/hcp/thcp_dorlands_content.jsp.
4. ThinkExist Quotations, http://en.thinkexist.com/quotation/next_to_love-sympathy_is_the_divinest_passion_of/175331.html (accessed February 1, 2007).
5. http://www.aafp.org/fpm/970400fm/lead.html#1.
6. Stress Less, http://www.stressless.com (accessed February 1, 2007).
7. Frampton, Gilpin, and Charmel, *Putting Patients First*, 6.
8. Childre and Cryer, *From Chaos to Coherence*, 69.
9. Ibid.

CHAPTER 7: WHEN IT'S HARD TO FOCUS

1. Teresa Gallagher, Born to Explore!, http://borntoexplore.org/neurochem.htm (accessed February 1, 2007).
2. Katrina Berne, PhD, Running on Empty (Alameda, CA: Hunter House, 1995), 58–59.
3. Ibid., 212.
4. Cyber Nation International, The People's Cyber Nation, http://cybernation.com/victory/quotations/authors/quotes_mandino_og.html (accessed February 1, 2007).

CHAPTER 8: FLOW INTO JOY!

1. Mihaly Csikszentmihalyi, Finding Flow: The Psychology of Engagement with Everyday Life (New York: Basic Books, 1998), 140.
2. Ibid., 34.
3. Bob Rotella, Golf Is Not a Game of Perfect (New York: Simon and Schuster, 1995), 77.
4. From an article titled "The Zone Demystified," provided to the author by Bruce Cryer, who helped found the Institute of HeartMath. According to Cryer, HeartMath is a well-developed system of tools, techniques, and technology backed by about fifteen years of scientific research. Part of what the practice of the HeartMath tools provides is a method for achieving "flow," on demand, when you need it. And their research helps people understand the biological underpinnings of what they are experiencing emotionally and spiritually. For further information about HeartMath, its products, and to view some of its research findings, visit Heartmath.com.
5. Csikszentmihalyi, Finding Flow, 49.

CHAPTER 9: THE ART OF PASTIME MANAGEMENT

1. Csikszentmihalyi, Finding Flow, 44.
2. American Cancer Society, "Humor Therapy: What Is It?" http://www.phoenix5.org/humor/HumorTherapyACS.html (accessed February 2, 2007).
3. Barry K. Baines, MD, Ethical Wills (New York: Perseus, 2002), 49–52.
4. Frampton, Gilpin, and Charmel, Putting Patients First, 137.
5. American Art Therapy Association, Inc., http://www.arttherapy.org/ (accessed February 2, 2007).
6. Frampton, Gilpin, and Charmel, Putting Patients First, 139–40.
7. American Music Therapy Association, "Frequently Asked Questions About Music Therapy," http://www.musictherapy.org/faqs.html#WHAT_IS_MUSIC_THERAPY.
8. Don Campbell, The Mozart Effect (New York: Avon, 1997), 243.

CHAPTER 10: A SACRED TIME

1. Joseph Martos, Doors to the Sacred (Liguori, MO: Liguori/Triumph, 2001), 18–19.

2. ThinkExist Quotations, http://en.thinkexist.com/quotation/each_day_is_a_special_gift_from_god-and_while/294618.html (accessed February 1, 2007).

CHAPTER 11: BOUNDARIES IN CAREGIVING
1. Cancer Treatment Centers of America, "Our Philosophy," http://www.cancer-center.com/about-us/philosophy.cfm (accessed February 1, 2007).
2. Daily Celebrations, http://www.dailycelebrations.com/joy.htm (accessed February 1, 2007).

CHAPTER 12: APPRECIATING OUR WAY INTO BETTER HEALTH
1. Rollin McCraty and Doc Childre, The Appreciative Heart (Boulder Creek, CA: HeartMath, n.d.), 5. HeartMath e-book.
2. Ibid., 6.
3. Ibid., 6–9.
4. Baker and Stauth, What Happy People Know, 37.
5. Ibid., 81.
6. Theodore Roosevelt Association, "In His Own Words," http://www.theodor-eroosevelt.org/life/quotes.htm (accessed February 1, 2007).
7. HeartMath LLC, HeartQuotes, http://www.heartquotes.net/Happiness.html (accessed February 1, 2007).

Additional copies of this and other
Life Journey products are available
wherever good books are sold.

Also available from Life Journey:
A Reason for Hope
A Season for Hope

If you have enjoyed this book,
or if it has impacted your life,
we would like to hear from you.

Please contact us at

LIFE JOURNEY
Cook Communication Ministries, Dept. 240
4050 Lee Vance View
Colorado Springs, CO 80918

Or visit our Web site
www.cookministries.com

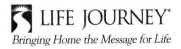

LIFE JOURNEY®
Bringing Home the Message for Life